Broiler meat inspection

For this English edition:

Broiler meat inspection

Plaza Antonio Beltrán Martínez nº 1, planta 8 - letra I
(Centro empresarial El Trovador)
50002 Zaragoza - Spain

First printing: July 2015

ISBN: 978-84-16315-28-4
D.L.: Z 1074-2015

Design, layout and printing:
Servet editorial - Grupo Asís Biomedia, S.L.
www.grupoasis.com
info@grupoasis.com

Warning:

Veterinary science is constantly evolving, as are pharmacology and the other sciences. Inevitably, it is therefore the responsibility of the veterinary clinician to determine and verify the dosage, the method of administration, the duration of treatment and any possible contraindications to the treatments given to each individual patient, based on his or her professional experience. Neither the publisher nor the author can be held liable for any damage or harm caused to people, animals or properties resulting from the correct or incorrect application of the information contained in this book.

EVILLE & JONES

Broiler
meat inspection

Antonio Lara Moreno

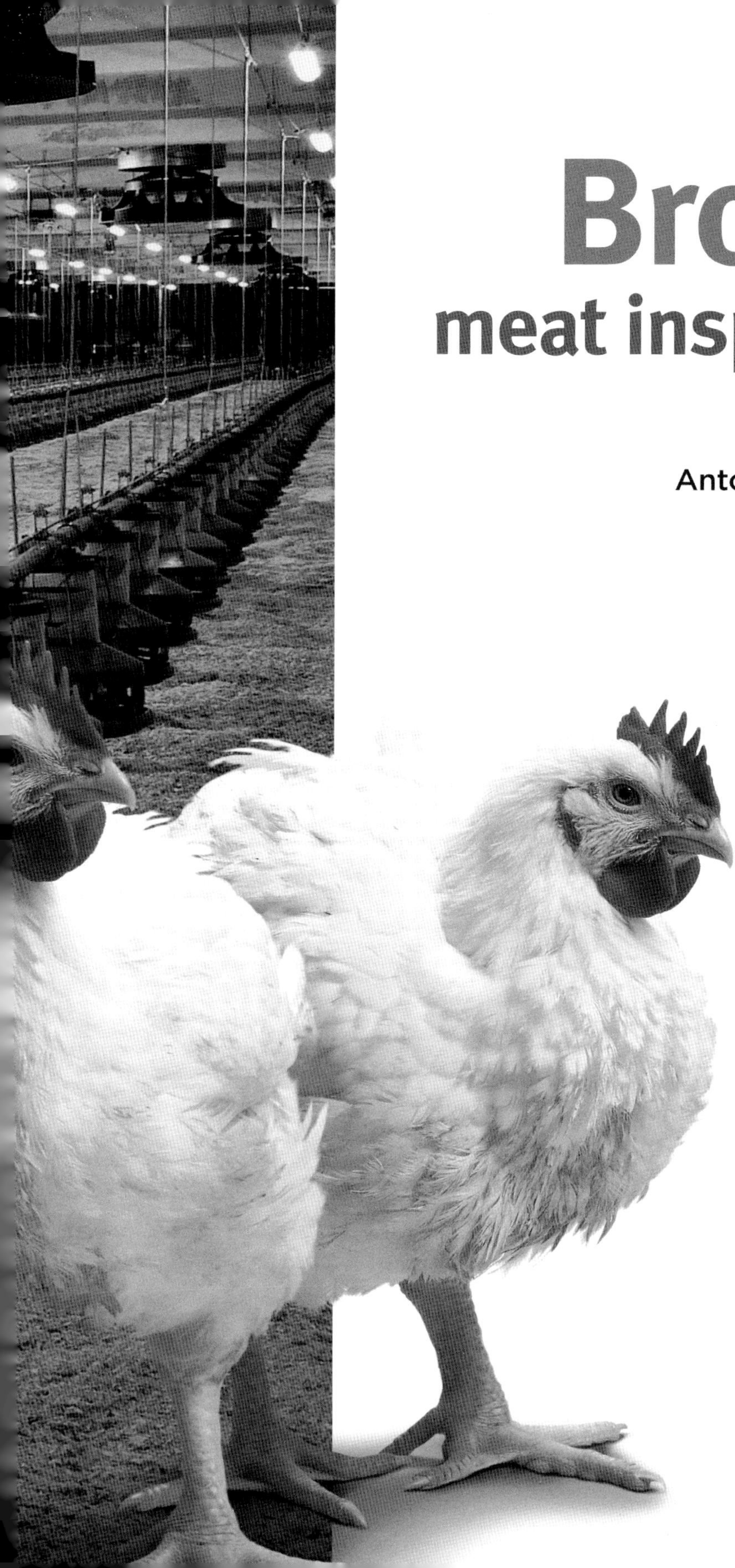

SERVET

To my beloved Alexandra
and my children Luis and Lola.

Acknowledgements

This photographic atlas would not have been possible without the support and help of many people. I honestly wish to express my gratitude to all meat inspectors and veterinarians who have contributed their time, dedication and knowledge.

My same gratitude goes to all abattoir personnel, without whose assistance, this work would not have been successful.

Finally, an honourable mention goes to my family and friends for their encouragement and support.

The author

Antonio Lara Moreno

He was awarded a degree in Veterinary Medicine from the University of Cordoba (Spain) and the Faculty of Veterinary Medicine of Maisons-Alfort (Paris, France) in 1998.

He is specialist in animal production and food hygiene, and acquired extensive professional experience in the UK since 1999 in the area of health inspection, particularly in the meat industry sector. Its main functions are focused on verifying the implementation of European Community legislation on animal and public health, with special attention to animal welfare and ante-mortem and post-mortem inspection of domestic animals for human consumption.

In 2001, he integrated the veterinary port inspection team of Southampton (England) in the control of animal products imported from third countries.

Between 2004 and 2013, he is specialised in the health inspection of poultry during slaughter in abattoirs.

Preface

This photographic atlas is intended for veterinary students, meat inspectors, farmers, and anyone in direct contact with the poultry industry. It is the result of years of dedication, research and experience as a veterinary inspector in poultry slaughterhouses.

The pictures reproduced in this work have all been taken during our day-to-day duties and they represent the most common conditions that can be found during the inspection of broilers at slaughter.

This work has been designed as a practical guide, easy to read and understand, yet an excellent tool for anyone involved in meat inspection of broilers and to a certain extent of other poultry species.

Author disclaimer

The content of this book is based on my own experience as a poultry veterinarian combined with literature, research and advice through consultation with others.

Antonio Lara Moreno

Table of contents

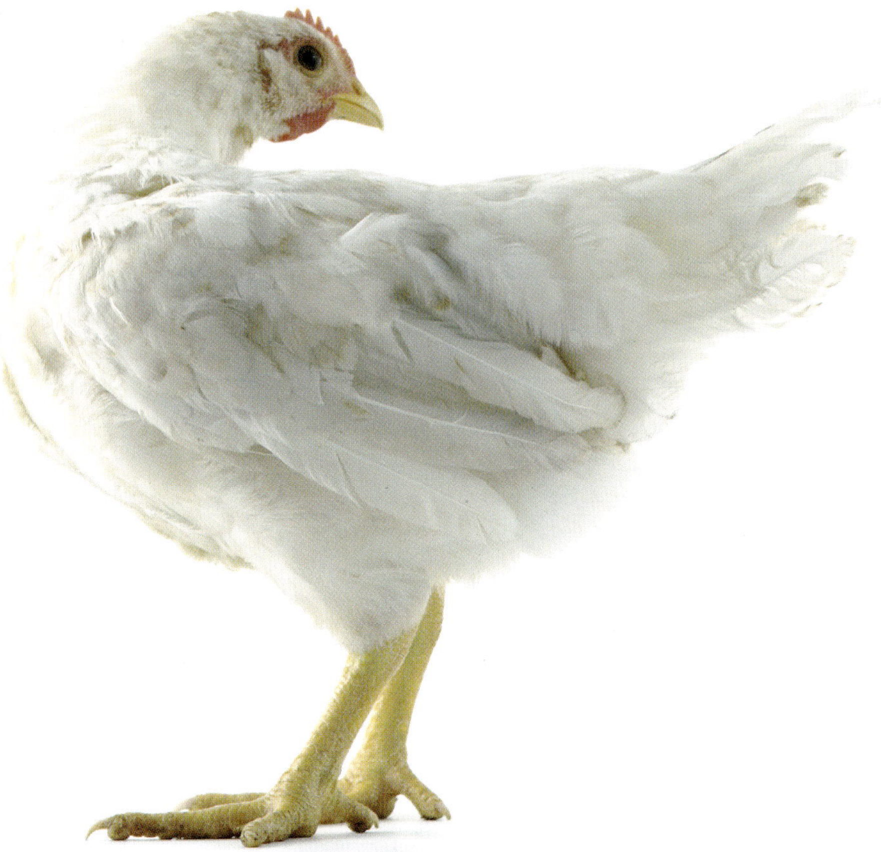

camellia/shutterstock.com

1

Introduction to poultry inspection

The inspection of poultry covers a wide range of controls aimed at ensuring that any meat unfit for human consumption is not allowed to progress into the food chain. Always refer to the current legislation in force when carrying out the duties as a veterinarian or inspector.

Food Business Operator Responsibilities

The primary responsibility of the Food Business Operator is to ensure that all stages of production result in a safe and wholesome product. Regulations outline some responsibilities of the establishment that are also specifically related to post-mortem inspection. These responsibilities include:

- Slaughtering poultry in accordance with good commercial practices.
- Sanitary practices in preparing the carcass for post-mortem inspection.
- Presenting carcasses and parts for inspection in a specified manner (called presentation).

The establishment's procedures to prepare poultry for inspection must take place in sanitary conditions and must use sanitary procedures to prevent contamination of the carcasses and parts. For example, during slaughter, the establishment must use sanitary dressing procedures to remove feathers and feet, open the carcasses, eviscerate, and shackle the carcasses.

The establishment must also ensure that the carcasses are presented for inspection in a specified manner. For example, each carcass must be opened to expose the organs and body cavity for proper examination by the inspector. They must also be hung on the line in a specified manner and spaced appropriately. The organs must be displayed in a specified order so that the inspector does not have to spend time locating them before he or she performs inspection procedures. Proper presentation helps to ensure consistent and accurate inspection. There are variations in the ways in which an establishment will present carcasses and parts for inspection. Veterinarians and inspectors will learn the specifics of presentation at the establishment where they are assigned. The proper presentation of carcasses for post-mortem inspection involves uniform and consistent feather removal, feet removal, opening of carcasses, evisceration, and shackling.

The establishment is also responsible for providing appropriate inspection stations that meet regulatory requirements. The requirements may vary depending on the size of the plant and volume of operations. For example, in large poultry slaughter establishments, there may be separate inspection stations for carcasses and for carcasses that are salvaged and reprocessed. However, if they are assigned to a very small plant, inspection for all of the regulatory requirements may take place in one location. The requirements also vary with the type of inspection system being used by the establishment.

Ante-mortem inspection

Ante-mortem inspection is performed on the day of slaughter by observing poultry in crates before or after removal from the lorries. When performing ante-mortem inspection the veterinarian or the inspector will pay attention to the following:

- The overall general condition of the birds, paying particular attention to the head, eyes and feet.
- Ante-mortem inspection must determine whether there is any sign that animal welfare has been compromised.
- The official veterinarian is to determine whether there is any condition which might adversely affect human or animal health, paying particular attention to the detection of zoonotic diseases and diseases on List A, where appropriate, and List B of the *Office International des Epizooties* (World Organization for Animal Health, OIE).

> **Signs of disease at ante-mortem inspection may include swelling of the head and eyes, oedema of the wattles, sneezing, abnormal coloured faeces or diarrhoea, lesions of the skin and bone or joint enlargement.**

Post-mortem inspection

Carcasses and accompanying offal are to be subjected without delay after slaughter to post-mortem inspection.

The general methods used when conducting on line poultry inspection involve the senses and are aimed to detect diseases, abnormalities and contamination. These include:

- **Sight:** observing a disease lesion (inflammatory process or tumour).
- **Feel:** palpating (feeling an abnormal lump or feeling abnormal firmness as an example).
- **Smell:** smelling decomposition, infection or toxins.

For detecting diseases and contamination it is needed to direct the attention to areas where they are likely to be found.

Diseases, abnormalities and contamination can occur at any place on the carcass or its parts. Signs of disease, abnormalities, and contamination will include variations in size, position, colour, shape, odour or consistency or a combination of these factors. Some of the diseases and abnormalities will produce visible or palpable lesions in specific locations. Remember that normal poultry carcasses will vary as a result of age, breed, gender, nutrition, management and slaughter practices. The firmness of the flesh and the colour and sheen of the tissues will depend on the age of the bird. The flesh and organ colour tones are generally brighter in younger birds. Colour tones tend to fade and decrease in intensity with advancing age. The comb and wattles of normal, commercially slaughtered birds may vary from bright red to pale red and even yellowish in colour.

When performing post mortem inspection, the veterinarian or the inspector will pay attention to the following:

1. **Observing the joints** for signs of inflammation, exudates or swelling which could indicate synovitis or arthritis.
2. **Observing the inside of the cavity** to look for any signs of inflammatory processes or presence of exudates which could indicate bacterial or viral infection, abnormal tissue masses or tumours, etc.
3. **Examination of the viscera** to look for any abnormality in size or colour of the organs, general congestion and signs of inflammation or infection.
4. **Examination of the outside of the carcass** could reveal skin lesions, general wasted condition of the carcass and abnormal colour. Poorly bled carcasses, overscalded carcasses with a cooked appearance and feet lesions such as pododermatitis or hock burn will also be looked for.
5. The inspector will **classify any unfit material** into the relevant by-product category in accordance with the relevant legislation in force and the Food Business Operator's procedures.
6. The inspector must ensure that **legal requirements for recording and reporting results** are followed accurately, and that the Food Business Operator is informed of unusual conditions or conditions that occur in significant numbers.

The purpose of post-mortem inspection is to make a judgement about the wholesomeness of each poultry carcass inspected. One of the following outcomes will result from post-mortem inspection:

- If the carcass is wholesome without any localised disease condition, it is passed as fit for human consumption. If it does have a localised condition the carcass would be trimmed by the inspector's helper or a trimmer. Removed parts are considered to be inedible and are condemned. The remainder of the carcass, which is now wholesome or free of disease, is allowed to continue after removal of the affected areas to become fit for human consumption. Carcasses may be passed subject to salvage or reprocessing at an offline station.
- If a final decision cannot be made by the inspector, the carcass will be detained for further examination. The identity of these carcasses must be maintained until a final examination has been completed. The veterinarian reviews all such carcasses and makes a final disposition of whether to pass, trim or condemn the bird.
- If there are systemic signs that indicate the carcass is unwholesome or diseased, the entire carcass is condemned.

2

Animal welfare

Definition

> **Animal welfare covers a very wide range of aspects aimed at avoiding unnecessary suffering to animals and to make sure that their production is controlled and maintained to acceptable levels of comfort and humanity.**
>
> **Always refer to current legislation in force. Legislation is constantly undergoing changes by means of amendments, repeals and other modifications.**

Broilers need to be looked after so that their welfare needs are properly met in accordance with the relevant animal welfare regulations.

The European Legislation lays down minimum rules to protect chickens kept and reared for meat production. In this chapter it will start covering the minimum requirements to be met at the farm in relation to the animal welfare of live birds.

In addition to the relevant provisions of other relevant community legislation, the following requirements shall apply:

1. Drinkers shall be positioned and maintained in such a way that spillage is minimised.
2. Feed shall be either continuously available or be meal fed and must not be withdrawn from chickens more than 12 hours before the expected slaughter time.
3. All chickens shall have permanent access to litter that is dry and friable on the surface.
4. Ventilation shall be sufficient to avoid overheating and, where necessary, in combination with heating systems to remove excessive moisture.
5. The sound level shall be minimised. Ventilation fans, feeding machinery or other equipment shall be constructed, placed, operated and maintained in such a way that they cause the least possible amount of noise.
6. All buildings shall have lighting with an intensity of at least 20 lux during the lighting periods, measured at bird eye level and illuminating at least 80 % of the useable area. A temporary reduction in the lighting level may be allowed when necessary following veterinary advice.
7. Within seven days from the time when the chickens are placed in the building and until three days before the foreseen time of slaughter, the lighting must follow a 24-hour rhythm and include periods of darkness lasting at least six hours in total, with at least one uninterrupted period of darkness of at least four hours, excluding dimming periods.

8. All chickens kept on the holding must be inspected at least twice a day. Special attention should be paid to signs indicating a reduced level of animal welfare and/or animal health.
9. Chickens that are seriously injured or show evident signs of health disorder, such as those having difficulties in walking, severe ascites or severe malformations, and are likely to suffer, shall receive appropriate treatment or be culled immediately. A veterinarian shall be contacted whenever necessary.
10. Those parts of buildings, equipment or utensils which are in contact with the chickens shall be thoroughly cleaned and disinfected every time after final depopulation is carried out, before a new flock is introduced into the house. After the final depopulation of a house, all litter must be removed, and clean litter must be provided.
11. The owner or keeper shall maintain a record for each house of a holding of:
    - The number of chickens introduced.
    - The useable area.
    - The hybrid or breed of the chickens, if known.
    - By each control, the number of birds found dead with an indication of the causes, if known, as well as the number of birds culled with cause.
    - The number of chickens remaining in the flock following the removal of chickens for sale or for slaughter.
12. All surgical interventions carried out for reasons other than therapeutic or diagnostic purposes which result in damage to or the loss of a sensitive part of the body or the alteration of bone structure shall be prohibited. However, beak trimming may be authorised by Member States when other measures to prevent feather pecking and cannibalism are exhausted. In such cases, it shall be carried out only after consultation and on the advice of a veterinarian and shall be carried out by qualified staff on chickens that are less than 10 days old. In addition, Member States may authorise the castration of chickens. The castration shall only be carried out under veterinary supervision by personnel who have received a specific training.

There are other requirements in relation to stocking density per square meter and record keeping which may also affect the welfare of animals, please refer to relevant legislation for more details.

Origin

The five freedoms of animal welfare

The Farm Animal Welfare Council (FAWC) - a government advisory body - has established five freedoms for animal welfare. These state that, at all times, it is had a duty of care to ensure that the animals are free:

- **From hunger and thirst** - animals must have access to fresh water and a diet which will maintain health and vigour.
- **From discomfort** - an appropriate environment should be provided, including shelter and a comfortable resting area.
- **From pain, injury or disease** - it must be ensured the prevention of illnesses, or rapid diagnosis and treatment.
- **To express normal behaviour** - sufficient space, proper facilities and company of the animal's own kind should all be provided.
- **From fear and distress** - it must be provided conditions and treatment which avoid mental suffering.

Animal welfare breaches may develop due to very numerous factors during production on farms, transport to the abattoir or during processing. Both the veterinarian and the inspector shall try to establish the cause of such breaches so they can be avoided in the future and reported accordingly (Fig. 1). This chapter will focus mainly on factors that can create a potential animal welfare problem during processing.

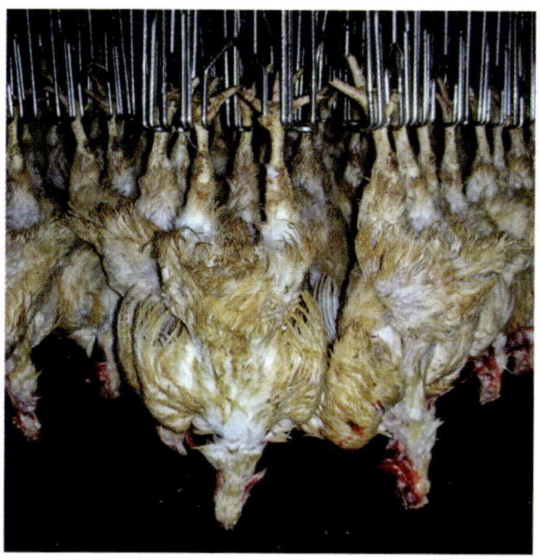

FIGURE 1. The veterinarian or inspector shall verify cleanliness and general condition of the birds at ante-mortem inspection and enforce any animal welfare concerns accordingly.

The most common **causes of animal welfare problems at the farm** could be listed as follows:

- Poor management practices.
- Poor bedding quality or inadequate bedding management.
- High density of birds per m² in the sheds.
- Poor ventilation.
- Bad management of the ambient temperature, humidity, light intervals and nutrition.
- Bacterial, viral and parasite diseases (vaccination ineffective).

Animal welfare issues during transport (Figs. 2 and 3) may be due to:

- An excessive number of birds per crate during transportation to the abattoir.
- Poor maintenance of crates and modules or any other transport means.
- Excessive duration of transport/distance to the abattoir.
- Ineffective protection against weather adversities, depending on the time of year, mainly against rain, heat and cold.
- Ineffective means of ventilation during transport.

Finally, the **most common causes of an animal welfare problem at the abattoir** may be listed as follows:

- Inadequate lairage in terms of noise level, protection against adverse weather, ventilation levels, temperature control, careful handling of modules/crates and maintenance of equipment.
- Excessive waiting time between arrival and the slaughter process, particularly during warm and cold weather.
- Bad handling of live birds at hanging point. Insufficient training given to personnel. Careless and violent behaviour at hanging point by relevant personnel.
- Poor maintenance of shackles. Damaged shackles can cause injury to live birds during the hanging process and they can also compromise the stunning, killing and bleeding process. Birds hanging by one leg may be at risk of receiving pre-stun shocks during stunning, furthermore, they are likely to miss the neck cutter when used and suffer cuts to the wings.
- Inappropriate length of time between hanging on and the stunning process. It is important to note that this interval can be affected during breakdowns and by a slow speed of the line. Always refer to current legislation to ensure that such requirements are met (not more than 2 minutes for broilers under the European legislation). During long breakdowns of the automated line, birds shall be taken off the line and put back into the crates to avoid any unnecessary stress.

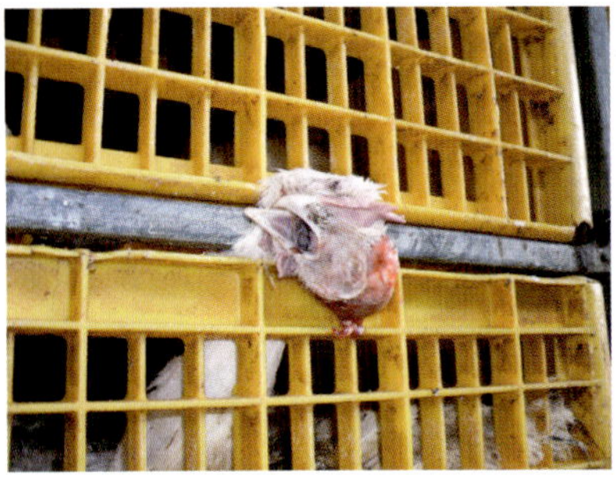

FIGURE 2. This incident was referred for investigation when identified during ante-mortem inspection.

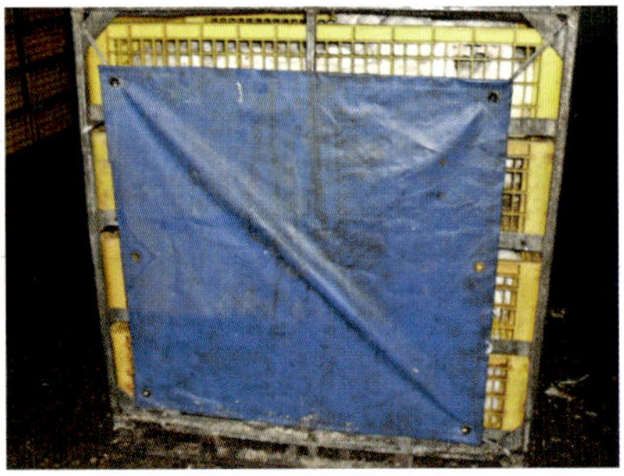

FIGURE 3. Lateral protection of the modules during transport used with very low outside temperatures.

- Ineffective stunning of birds. This can be caused by improper setting of the stunner, poorly maintained or faulty stunner or due to improper adjustment of the height of the stunning bath (in relation to bird's size).
- Water bath pre-stun shocks. Pre-stun shocks are due to inconsistencies between the design of the stunner bath, its proper height adjustment and the size of the bird being slaughtered. Pre-stun shocks are produced when parts of the birds, particularly wings, touch the electrified water before the head enters the water and effective stunning is produced.
- Ineffective neck cutter or killing machine when used. Poor maintenance as well as improper adjustment of the automatic neck cutter may lead to birds missing the neck cutter as well as birds not being effectively slaughtered. Insufficient neck cutting will compromise the bleeding process.
- Bad/insufficient bleeding. This could be due to a malfunction of the neck cutter or its improper adjustment and it increases the chances of birds entering the scalding tanks still alive. It is paramount to allow sufficient bleeding time so such a scenario is avoided in all cases (bleeding times are normally more than two minutes). Current European legislation requires a minimum bleeding time of 90 seconds for broilers.
- Birds missing the neck cutter following stunning. When head only stunning or electronarcosis is used, electric current is given to the head of the animal causing a disruption of the brain's activity which renders the bird unconscious. Birds that for some reason miss the neck cutter and bleeding is not produced will regain consciousness before entering the scalding tank alive. These birds are commonly known as "uncut birds" and they can be easily identified at post-mortem inspection (Fig. 4).
- Other stunning methods may include electrocution and subsequent death due to cardiac arrest, and although it delivers better welfare results, some operators choose not to use it claiming that it produces damage to the carcass and bad bleeding (blood spots and fractures).

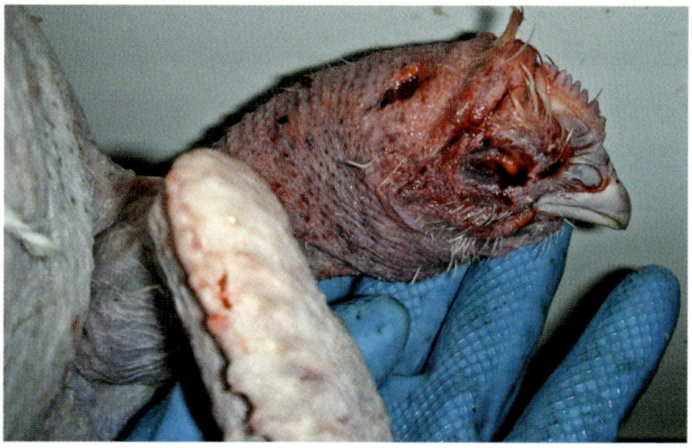

FIGURE 4. Uncut bird to show no signs of cutting of the neck and congestion of the head. This particular incident was referred for investigation.

Responsibilities

> Safeguarding animal welfare is one of the most important roles to be performed by the veterinarian and the inspector. Any situation in which the welfare of animals is thought to be compromised shall require immediate action in order to avoid unnecessary suffering of the affected animals, particularly if the suffering is being produced during the slaughter process. Any signs which may indicate an animal welfare problem at the farm of origin shall be reported to the competent authority for possible investigation. The inspector is therefore a key element in the enforcement of animal welfare legislation.

According to the European legislation, those involved in the management of birds for slaughter should be trained according to their responsibilities.

During **ante-mortem inspection**, the veterinary inspector shall verify that:

1. The construction and design of the reception area modules provides good protection against inclement weather. They should be large enough to accommodate a number of modules that depend on the production volume of the slaughterhouse.
2. The maintenance of the baskets and transport modules should not jeopardize the integrity of the birds during transport or during the transfer process to the production line. The Food Business Operator should have a system in place to monitor the maintenance of the crates/modules and their repair or replacement when needed (Fig. 5).

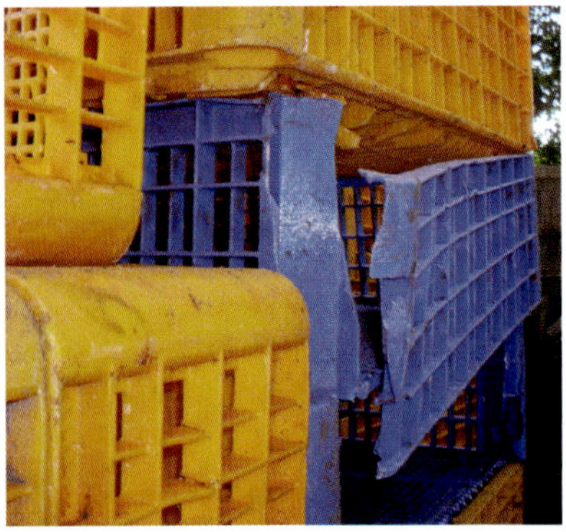

FIGURE 5. Broken crates being removed for recycling.

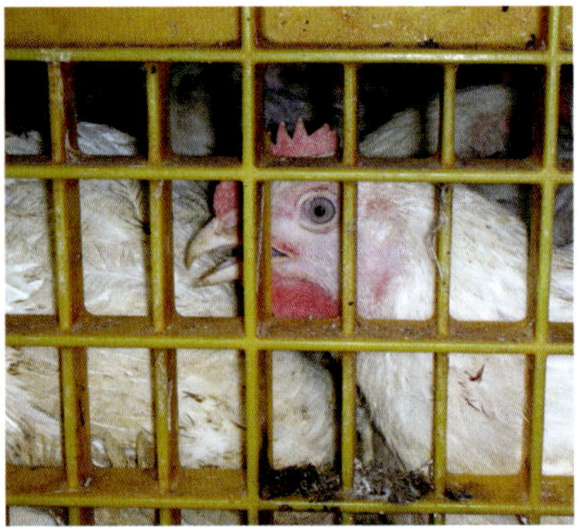

FIGURE 6. Panting is common in summer hot days.

3. The density of birds per basket must be appropriate considering the weather conditions (outside temperature) and the size of the animals. Other factors to consider are the time before slaughter and ventilation systems in the slaughterhouse. The waiting time before slaughter should be as small as possible to decrease subsequent death by suffocation, particularly in summer days. The modules should be protected from direct sunlight and forming corridors with enough separation for adequate ventilation. The use of fans is recommended for ventilation of the modules when the outside temperature is above 15 degrees. In our experience, the most frequent cause of death before slaughter derives from inadequate control of the procedures mentioned in this section. Birds do not have sweat glands to dissipate heat, their only means of dissipation is through expired air, and if it is added that their bodies are covered with feathers, not surprisingly, an increase of several degrees centigrade in body temperature means death by suffocation.
4. During the ante-mortem inspection, the veterinary inspector certifies the integrity of the animals and their overall health, paying particular attention to the following:
    - Breathing abnormalities.
    - Signs of ocular congestion.
    - Discolouration of the comb and wattles.
    - Presence of exudates in eyes and nostrils.
    - State of the feathers.
    - Cleanliness and general condition of the birds.
    - Uneven sizes paying particular attention to runts and emaciated birds.
    - Presence of dermatitis and pododermatitis.
    - Density per basket in relation to the size of the birds and the outside temperature (Fig. 6).
    - Signs of stress.
5. The veterinarian or inspector will also verify that the transfer of the animals to the production line is carried out without causing unnecessary stress to the animals and that the personnel involved in the transfer have received the necessary training. Excessive noise in the surrounding areas prior to the transfer to the production line can also be a stress factor for birds. Relevant checks will follow to verify that pre-stun shocks do not occur during the stunning.

All birds leaving the waterbath stunner must be checked by the Food Business Operator to ensure they have been effectively stunned or killed. If a stun is effective, and the bird is unconscious post-stun, it will show the following signs:

- No rhythmic breathing for 10-20 seconds after leaving the waterbath.
- Neck arched with head directed vertically.
- Dilated pupils.
- Absence of a corneal or third eyelid response.
- No reaction to comb pinch.
- Wings held close to the body.
- Rigidly extended legs (not an appropriate indicator when a bird is held in a shackle).
- Constant body tremors (movement).

If the stun is ineffective, the bird may show the following signs:

- Return of rhythmic breathing.
- A corneal or third eyelid response.
- Tension in the neck muscles.
- Other voluntary muscle movements.
- Vocalisation.

If the bird has received an effective stun/kill, and it is dead, the following signs will be seen:

- Fixed, central, dilated pupils.
- No rhythmic breathing.
- No response to any stimuli e.g. no corneal or third eyelid response or reaction to comb pinch.
- Limp carcass.
- There will be no body tremors or movement.

During **post-mortem inspection** the veterinarian or inspector will supplement ante-mortem inspection by detecting any lesions that are relevant to animal welfare. The official veterinarian shall evaluate the results of the post-mortem inspection to identify possible indications of poor welfare conditions such as abnormal levels of contact dermatitis, parasitism and systemic illness. If the mortality rate or the results of the post-mortem inspection are consistent with poor animal welfare conditions, the official veterinarian shall communicate the data to the owner or keeper of the animals and to the competent authority. Appropriate actions shall be taken by the owner or the keeper of the animals and by the competent authority.

3
Congenital malformations

Definition

Congenital malformations are anomalies that occur during the development of the chicken resulting in structural and/or functional abnormalities.

> **Most malformations found in broilers during routine inspection affect the skeletal system. The most frequent ones according to author's experience are supernumerary and/or deformed limbs.**

Less frequent deformities may affect the structure, number and colouration of feathers. Heart and ocular malformations are also possible but they are not easily identifiable at post-mortem inspection point. The same applies to malformations of the gastrointestinal as well as the urogenital system which, although they have been confirmed, they are of very little relevance while carrying out post-mortem inspection.

Congenital malformations in general are rare but well known within the poultry industry.

Cause/Origin

The cause of the majority of animal malformations is unknown, although it is thought that a significant proportion of congenital malformations of unknown cause are likely to have an important genetic component.

Deformities of the spine have been reported in poultry birds. Most of these reports describe **scoliosis**, a malformation of multiple aetiology including primarily genetic factors (improper differentiation of spinal segments).

Polymelia is a birth defect involving limbs in which the affected bird has more than the usual number of limbs. The external features show two normal limbs plus one or more undeveloped, extra-limbs (Figs. 1

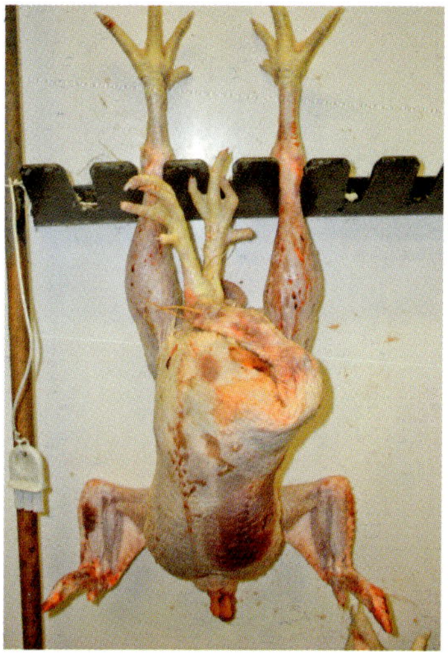

FIGURE 1. Polymelia to show two undeveloped extra limbs.

and 2). These are normally attached to the caudal region of the pelvic bone and surrounded by a mass of muscular tissue (Fig. 3). Also, they appear to be formed at a joint with the pelvis, presenting a characteristic incompletely duplicated femur and tibia. According to different studies, congenital malformations of the limbs are among the most frequent congenital anomalies found in animals and humans. However, the precise mechanism that regulates their development is not yet clearly understood. These anomalies are usually associated with genetic factors including trans-genes, chromosomes, and environmental agents, toxins, techniques involved in fertilization and certain management factors or a combination of factors.

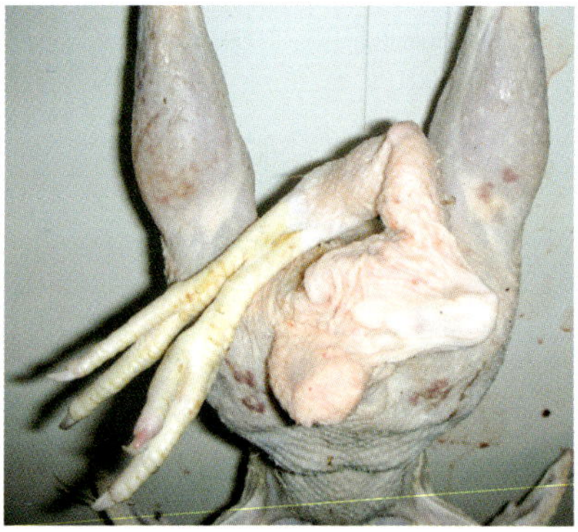

FIGURE 2. Polymelia. Two extra limbs.

Diplopodia is a congenital anomaly that involves duplication of elements of the foot on the hind limb (Fig. 4). Chickens normally have an anisodactyl toe arrangement, with one short toe pointing backwards and three long toes pointing forwards. In diplopodia, the feet usually lack the normal hind toe and instead develop two to four extra toes at various positions between the hock joint and the front toes. The toes are almost always connected to extra tarso-metatarsal bones, though sometimes the toes do not contain any bone.

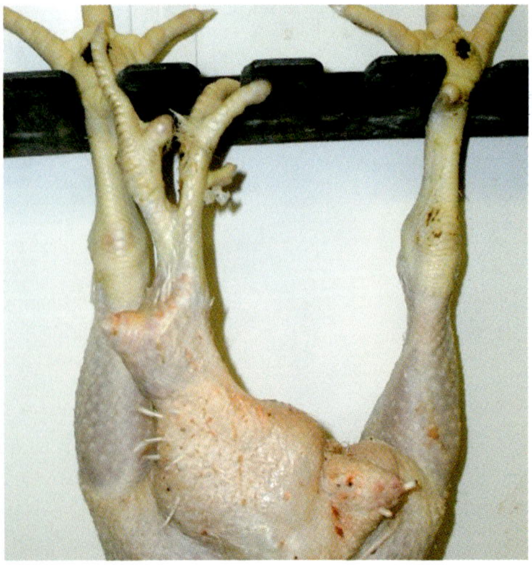

FIGURE 3. Polymelia to show two undeveloped extra limbs attached to the caudal region of the pelvic bone. This carcass was trimmed and eviscerated manually to avoid the risk of cross contamination and machine damage. Such carcasses are considered fit for human consumption and they will normally be sent to a cutting plant for further processing.

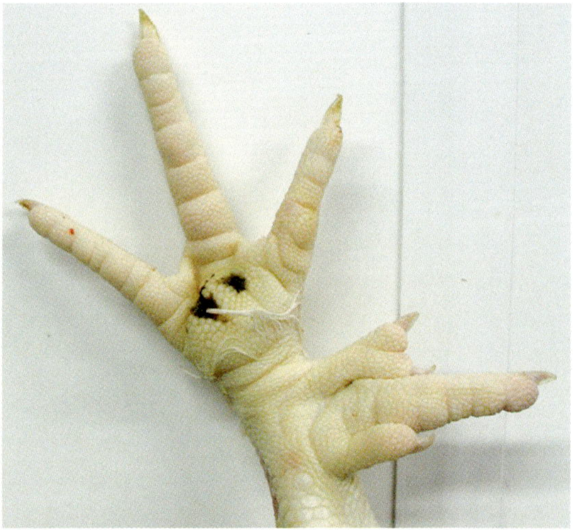

FIGURE 4. Classic diplopodia. Some extra digits attached to the metatarsus. The first normal digit that normally faces rearward is missing.

Responsibilities

In the vast majority of cases, removal of the deformity would be sufficient so that the rest of the carcass can be considered as fit for human consumption.

Certain malformations may contribute to poor or erratic evisceration and possible contamination, as well as machine damage, which could lead to a total condemnation of the carcass.

Congenital malformation sometimes leads to mortality, and it may also reduce the cost effectiveness and market value of defective birds. However, animals with supernumerary ectopic limbs can survive successfully with normal locomotion depending on the extent of the defect.

Most animals with congenital defects found at post-mortem inspection are in an apparently good state with no other anomalies observed. They normally reach slaughter weight without any other problems.

It is recommended to report such cases as this will add knowledge to the distribution of the defect. This will also facilitate the search for offending compounds in the environment and the eventual establishment of their causal relationships.

Image gallery of congenital malformations

A. Undeveloped phalanges of the first, second and third digit.

B. The carpometacarpal and the three digits of the wing are missing.

C. Rare extra digit attached to the skin only in the tibiotarsal region of both legs.

D. Undeveloped phalanges affecting all digits from one foot only. Claws have not developed.

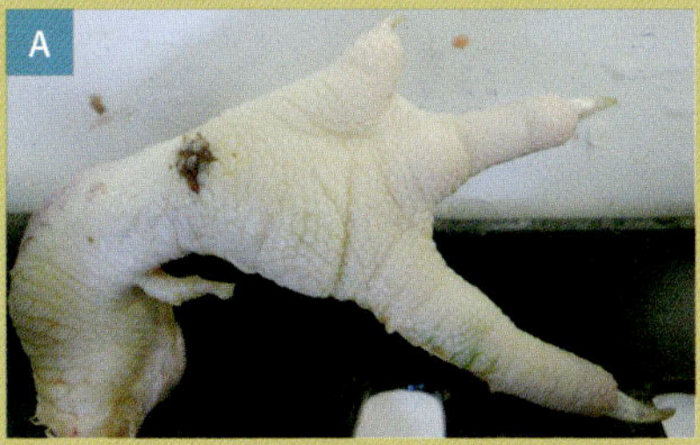

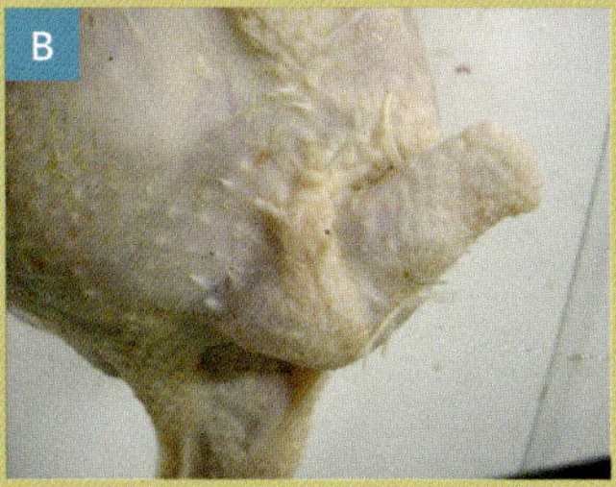

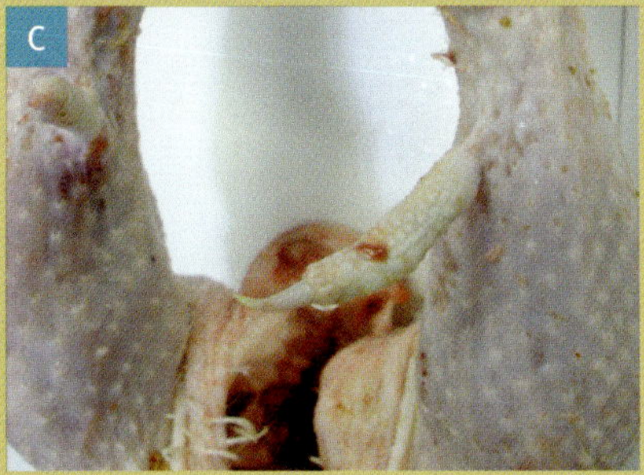

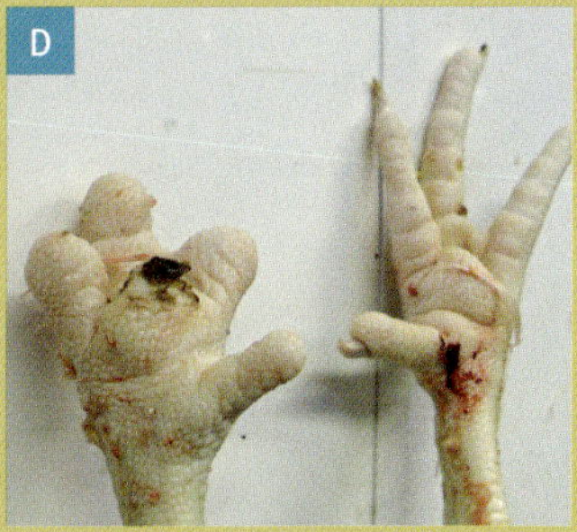

Image gallery of congenital malformations

E. Rare case of a carcass with two pygostyles.

F. Polymelia and rare presence of two cloacae.

G. Undeveloped or non-existent pygostyle.

H. Digestive abnormality in the form of an occlusion of the ileum. Carcasses are normally smaller in size but otherwise healthy. Such abnormalities of the digestive tract are rare and they represent a big risk of contamination during the evisceration process. Good general condition carcasses do not need to be condemned and they are passed as fit. Carcasses with extensive disruptions of the digestive functions like the one shown in this picture with signs of emaciation should be rejected. Birds that are undetected at whole bird inspection resulting in extensive machine damage or contamination during the evisceration process should also be discarded accordingly.

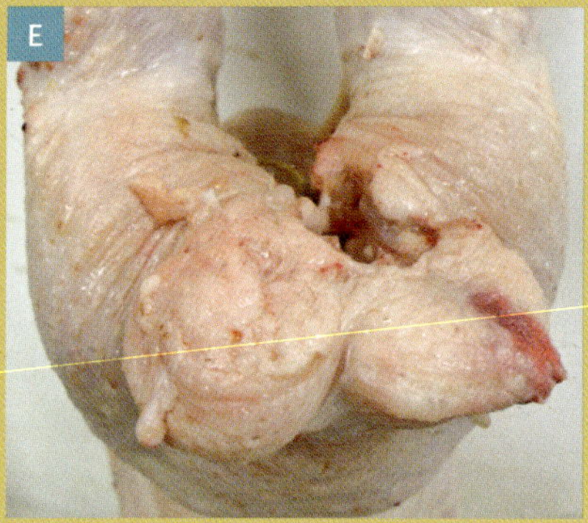

I. Malformation of the keel bone. Such condition is relatively frequent and it does not affect the wholesomeness of the carcass. The evisceration process is not normally affected. The carcass can be passed as fit for human consumption.

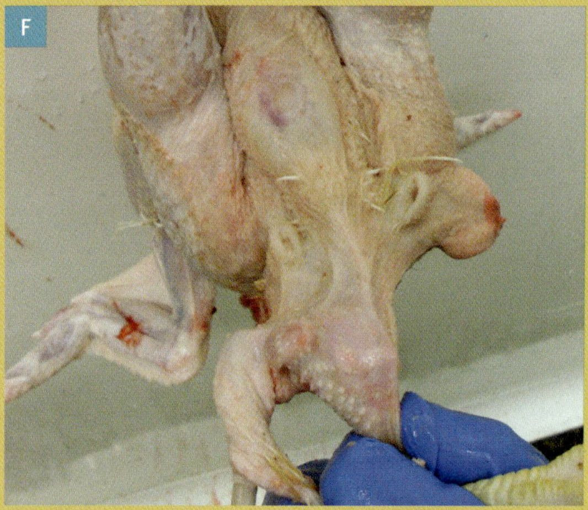

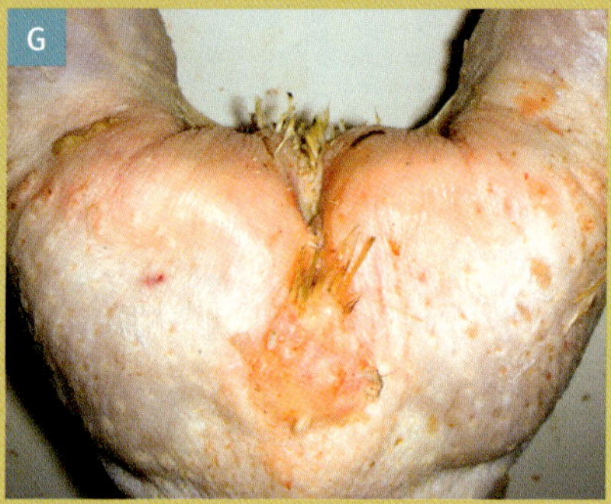

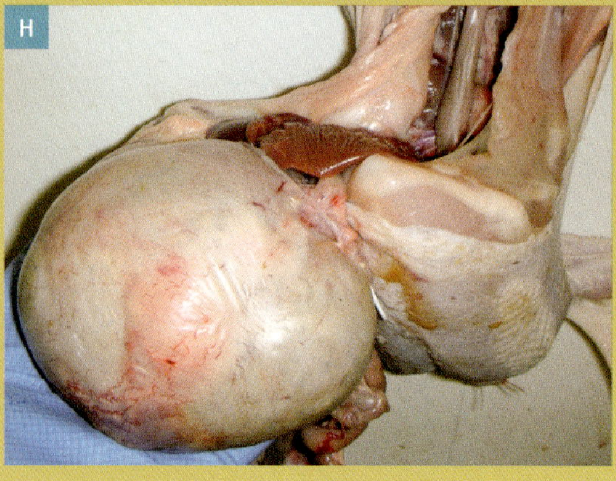

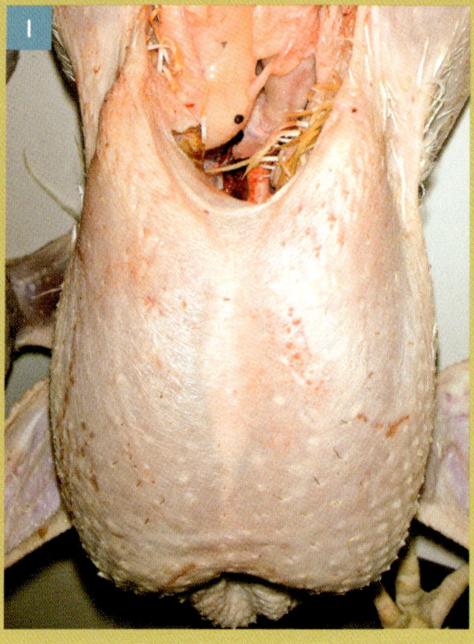

4

Arthritis, tenosynovitis and other joint lesions

Definition

Arthritis in broilers will normally affect the joints of the legs, usually the tibiometatarsal joint or hock joint (Fig. 1).

The synovial fluid is produced by the synovial cells that form the synovial membrane which is covered by a fibrous tissue forming the fibrous capsule. An inflammatory process of the joint increases the pressure causing deformities and degeneration of the articular cartilage. The spread of the infection to muscles and tendons can lead to **myositis** and **tenosynovitis**, respectively. When such inflammation only affects the subcutaneous tissue, it receives the name of **panniculitis**.

In the live bird, acute arthritis is characterised by an increase in volume, temperature and redness of the affected area. On palpation the consistency is soft.

The chronic form in a live bird is of a harder consistency with lesser temperature to the touch and smaller in size compared to an acute arthritis.

FIGURE 1. **Joint.**

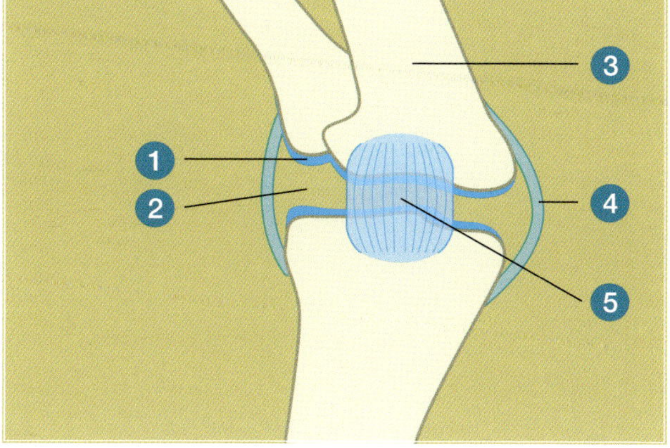

1. Articular cartilage.
2. Joint cavity filled with synovial fluid.
3. Bone.
4. Fibrous capsule.
5. Ligament.

Origin

The origin of arthritis and tenosynovitis in broilers can be very varied but generally classified as traumatic, infectious or toxic.

- **Traumatic arthritis** is the result of an injury that consequently triggers an inflammatory process and opens the door to potential secondary infections. As in most of the lesions detected during post-mortem inspection, it can never be ruled out an animal welfare problem at the farm in line with poor management, excessive density of birds per square meter, poor ventilation or poor bedding. Any of these factors may have a negative effect in the apparition of traumatic arthritis.
- **Infectious arthritis** can be caused by bacteria, viruses or a mixture of both. The most frequent viruses are usually reovirus, coronavirus and picornavirus. Bacterial infections frequently involve *Escherichia coli*, *Staphylococcus aureus*, *Streptococcus*, mycoplasmas, *Salmonella* and *Pasteurella*. With the exception of arthritis produced by mycoplasmas, which are usually serofibrinous, all other infections will generally produce a purulent arthritis. The most frequent primary causing agents are mycoplasmas and reovirus.
- **Toxic arthritis** is mostly related to uraemia or hyperuricaemia as a result of nephritis caused by a viral infection or due to inadequate protein diets.
- **Other leg problems** are due to genetic or nutritional source disorders and can be summarised as follows:
  - **Tibial dyschondroplasia**: due to the tibial cartilage not maturing enough to ossify leaving the growth plate prone to fracture, infection and deformed bone development. This condition is associated with excessive bone growth exceeding the bird's capacity to put calcium into the bone.
  - **Angular bone deformity**: occurs when the legs become bowed in or out, or twisted. It appears to be related to rapid growth with insufficient time for proper alignment and remodelling of the bones of the distal tibio-tarsus.
  - **Perosis**: produced due to deficiency of the trace minerals manganese and zinc and the vitamins choline, niacin, folic acid, biotine and pyridoxine. Symptoms include shortening and thickening of long bones, tibia and metatarsus bowing and lateral slipping of the achilles tendon.
  - **Spondylolistesis**: occurs when the ligaments between the third and fourth thoracic vertebrae tear or avulse and allow the anterior end of the fourth vertebrae to dislocate ventrally. The thoracic vertebrae T4 suffers a downward rotation, impinging on the spinal cord and causing leg weakness and ataxia. Affected birds will sit on their tail with their legs extended. Again, this condition is also related to fast bone growth and is also genetic related.
  - **Scoliosis**: congenital defect not associated with growth.

- **Rickets**: lack of mineralization of bones due to vitamin D, phosphorus or calcium deficiency. Vitamin D is the most common cause due to a mixing error in feed or toxins that interfere with normal metabolism. It causes deformities in legs and ribs with poor feather development and growth rate.

Responsibilities

Total or partial rejection of the carcass should be decided based on the extent of the injury of the affected joints (Fig. 2). Judgement is also made upon general condition of the carcass. Birds with leg problems are commonly found to be emaciated, dehydrated and septicaemic, in which case, a whole bird rejection is required. Trimming procedures, when applicable, will require removal of the affected part to the next healthy joint.

A high incidence of arthritis or leg problems, particularly if accompanied by other injuries such as footpad dermatitis, hock and breast burn or emaciation, must be notified to the competent authority for further investigation.

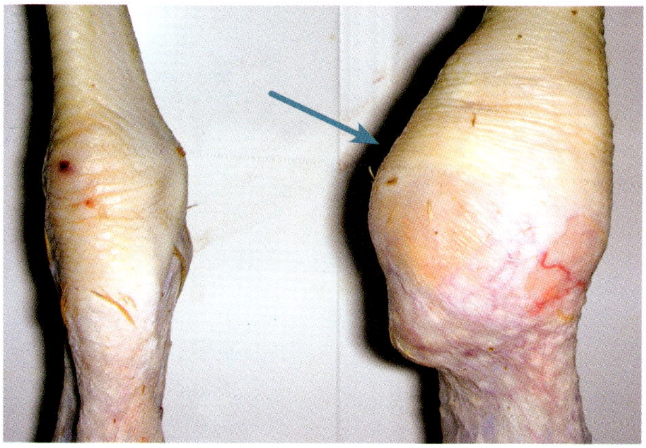

FIGURE 2. Localised joint lesion affecting only one joint.

> Leg problems in broilers have a huge impact in animal welfare. A painful lameness will reduce the bird's capability for movement which could result in starvation and dehydration to death.
>
> Leg problems may also increase the likelihood of hock and breast burns as a result of long periods of time in direct contact of the skin with the litter, as well as scratches by other birds, particularly during panic movements.

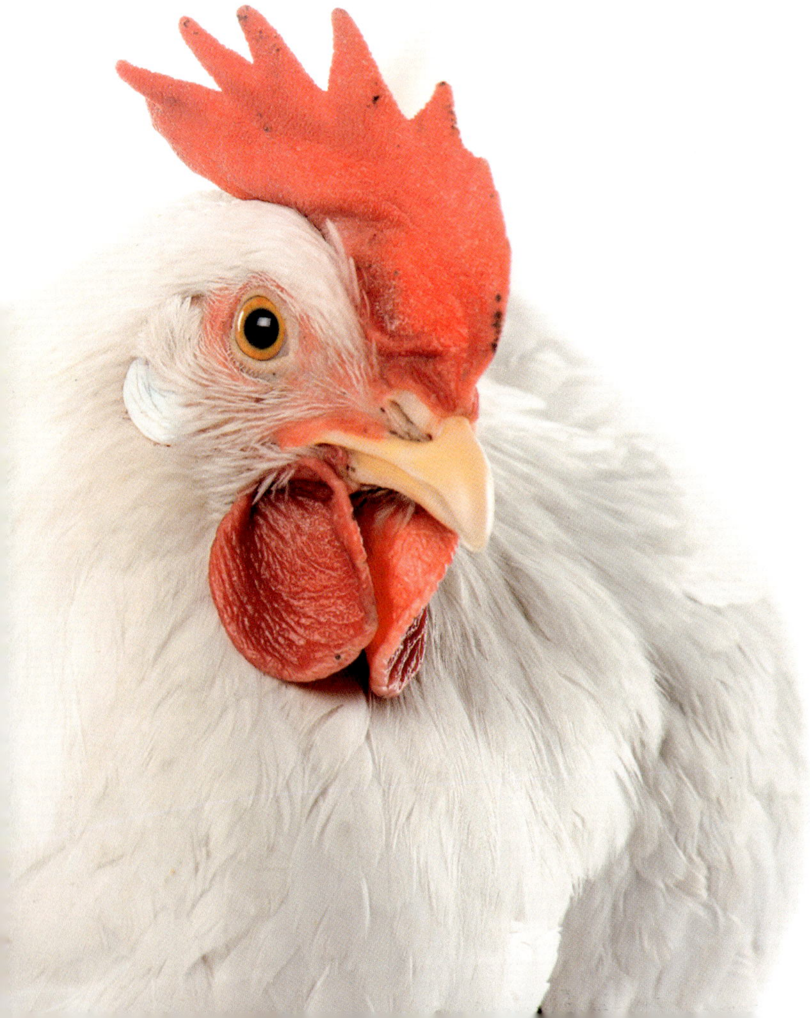

yevgeniy11/shutterstock.com

5

Cellulitis

Definition

Cellulitis is an infection of the connective tissue between the skin and the muscle, and it is normally found around the pericloacal area (Fig. 1), the thighs, lower abdomen and breast (Fig. 2). It is a seropurulent lesion accompanied by a thickening and a yellowing of the skin due to hyperkeratosis (Fig. 3).

> **Minor cellulitis is extremely difficult to detect at the inspection point and requires good concentration and years of experience. Many meat inspectors become skilled at detecting differences in skin colour in the affected birds.**

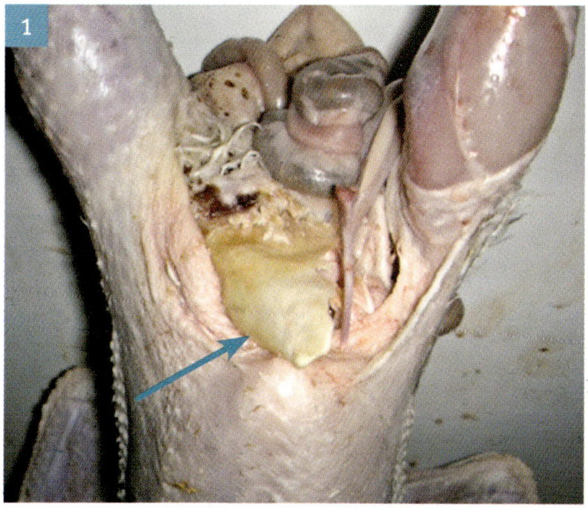

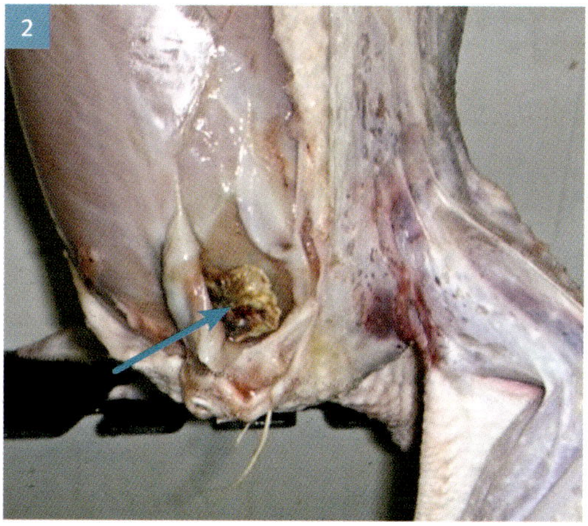

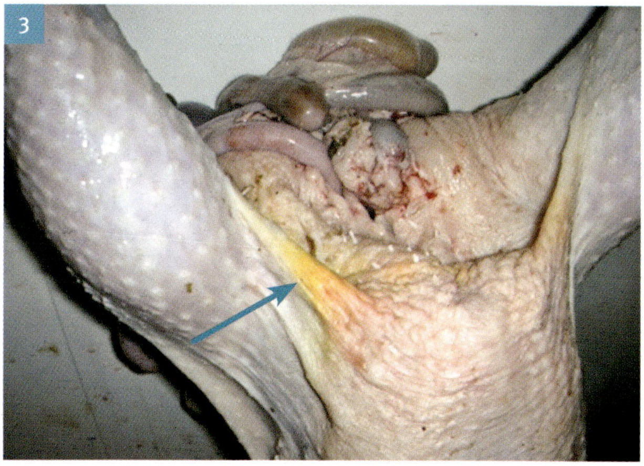

FIGURE 1. Dry form of cellulitis affecting pericloacal area. Total condemnation is recommended due to the extension of the infection under the skin.

FIGURE 2. Dry form of cellulitis affecting breast. Partial rejection possible.

FIGURE 3. Yellowing and thickening of the skin. Bilateral dry form of cellulitis.

There are two forms of cellulitis: a more common **dry form** (Fig. 4), and a **purulent form** that is normally associated with septicaemia.

The dry form is normally a localized lesion showing a sheet of dry pus underneath the skin and possible petechiae in the underlying muscles (Figs. 5 and 6).

The degree and extension of the lesion varies from one carcass to another.

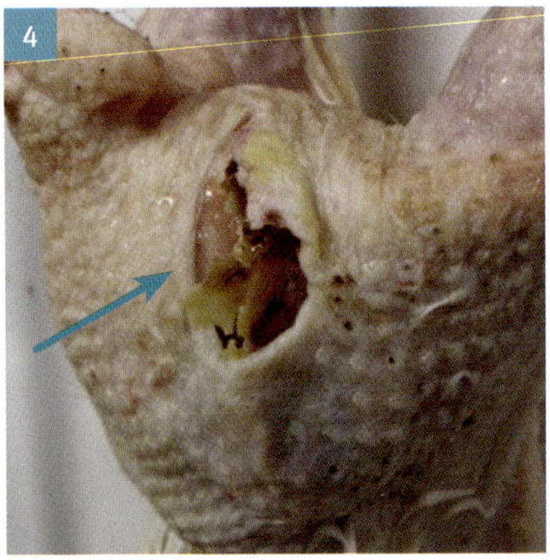

FIGURE 4. Cellulitis in its dry form. Note a sheet of dry pus underneath the skin. Also note the thickening and yellowing of the skin which should be the first indication for the inspector to suspect the presence of cellulitis.

FIGURE 5. Dry form of cellulitis revealing a sheet of pus and inflammation of the skin. Underlying muscles displaying small haemorrhages. Total condemnation of the carcass.

FIGURE 6. Dissection of the skin to reveal a soft sheet of pus turning into a dry form of cellulitis.

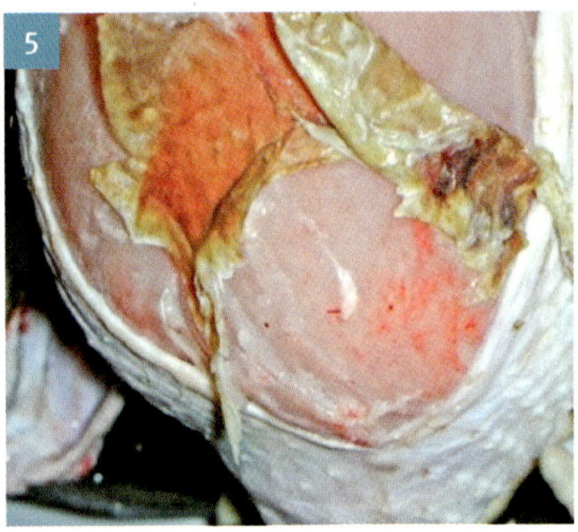

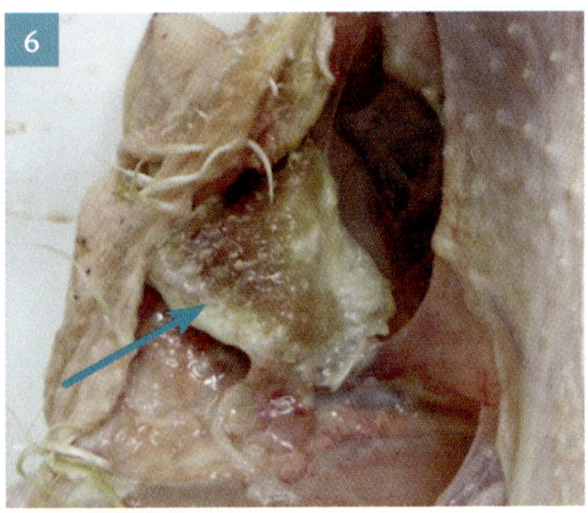

Origin

The origin of cellulitis is, according to author's experience, a mere combination of several factors. The lesion is initially started by a scratch that becomes infected.

The anatomy of modern broiler plays an important role since a very prominent and poorly feathered abdomen increases the chance of scratches.

Management skills at the farm are always related to the level of pathological conditions within the flock, for example, clean well managed bedding not only decreases the chance of scratches but also maintains a low and acceptable level of bacterial contamination. The control of the temperature in the sheds in intensive broiler production plays an important role in the feathering development and consequently in the incidence of cellulitis.

> The connective tissue under the skin will get infected in line with the level of bacterial contamination of the environment. For example, a humid litter favouring the bacterial multiplication will increase the likelihood of cellulitis.
>
> *E. coli* is normally the causing agent and most frequently isolated.

The density of birds within the flock is obviously a risk factor in that a more nervous flock will favour scratches, hence a potential increase in the level of cellulitis.

Responsibilities

Total or partial condemnation of the carcass will need to be accessed upon extension and nature of the lesion (Fig. 7). Small localized cellulitis in its dry form may be trimmed in those cases where no other conditions are observed and when the carcass is in good general condition. Whole bird rejection is the most sensible approach in the case of cellulitis in its wet form (Fig. 8), and when lesions are not localized (Fig. 9).

In the vast majority of cases the carcass is discarded due to the risk of cross contamination during the trimming procedures (Figs. 10 and 11) and considering that *E. coli* is the most frequent causative organism (Fig. 12).

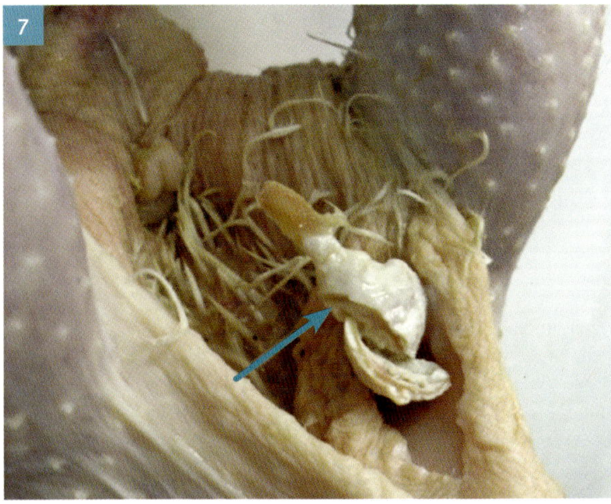

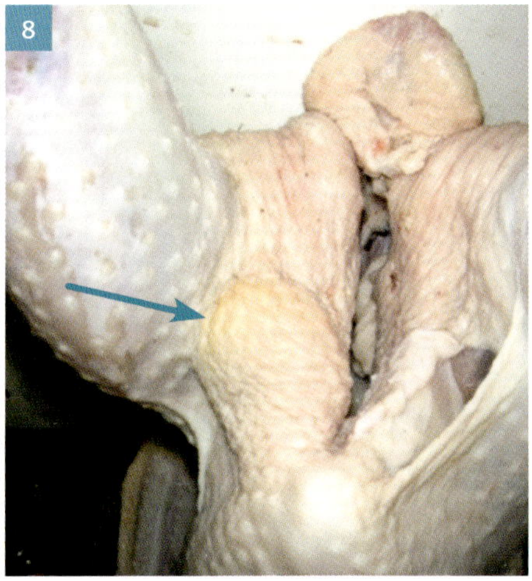

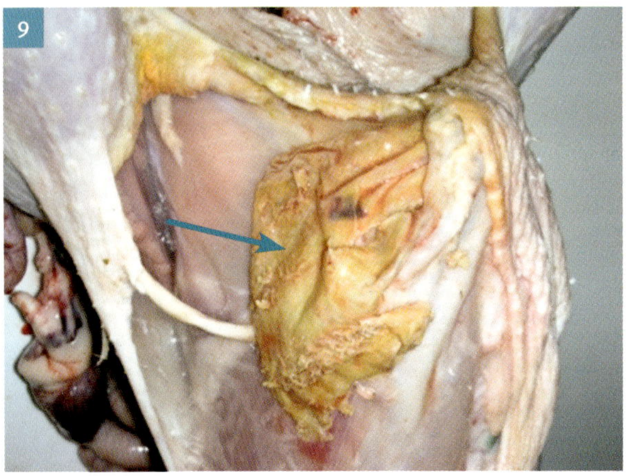

FIGURE 7. Caseous cheeselike cellulitis. Trimming may be considered.

FIGURE 8. Unilateral wet form of cellulitis. Note the yellowing and thickening of the skin. This condition is found more frequently in older broilers (45 to 60 days old). The inflammation and hyperkeratosis makes the condition more noticeable and therefore easier to detect at the inspection point.

FIGURE 9. Incision of the skin to show dry sheet of pus. Total condemnation of the carcass due to the extension of the lesion across the breast muscles.

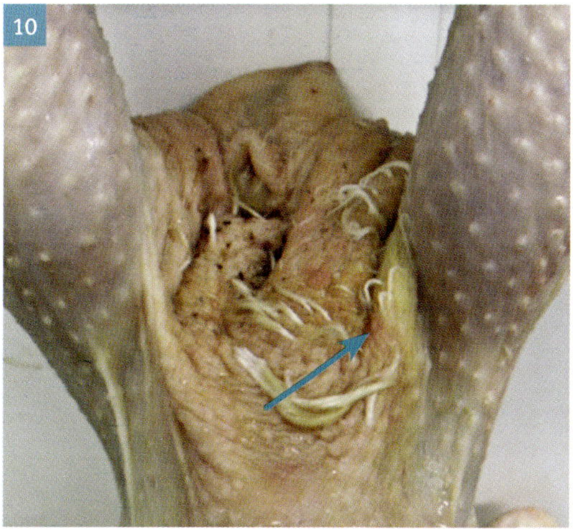

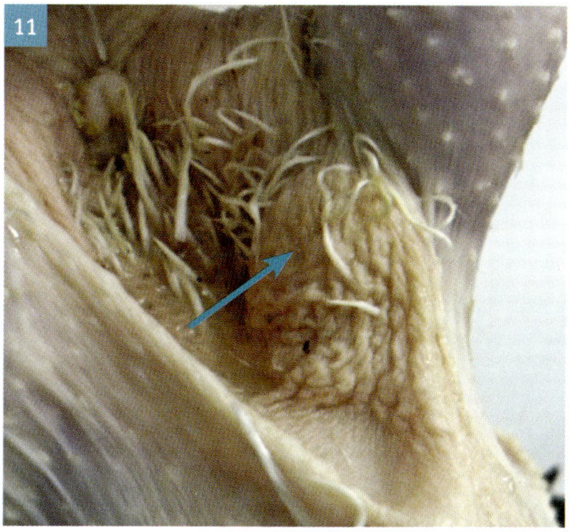

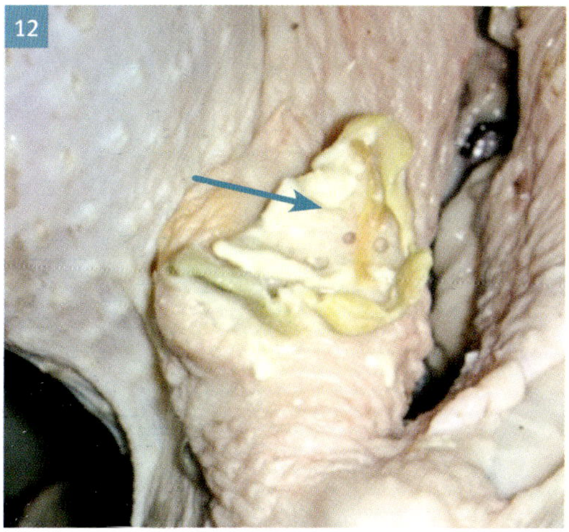

FIGURE 10. Yellowing and thickening of the skin to indicate potential presence of infection at whole bird inspection point.

FIGURE 11. Skin lump easy to detect during whole bird inspection, hard to the touch indicating presence of infection.

FIGURE 12. Dissection of the affected skin to show deposits of yellowish caseous pus. Total carcass condemnation due to the risk of cross contamination (*E. coli*).

A high prevalence of cellulitis, especially if accompanied by other conditions such as pododermatitis or breast burn, will need to be considered by the meat inspector as an indicative of a potential animal welfare problem.

Those cases will need to be reported to the competent authority for further investigation at the farm when necessary.

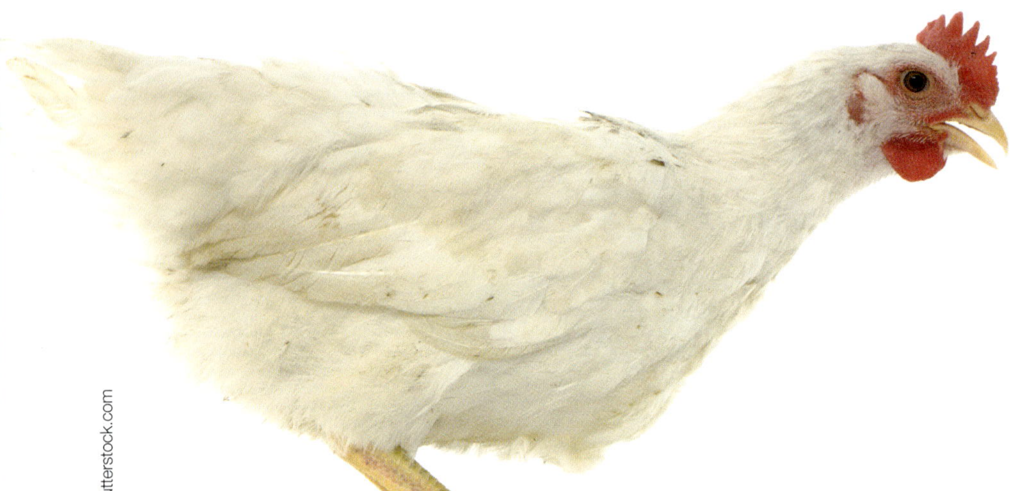

camellia/shutterstock.com

6

Dermatitis and pododermatitis

Definition

In this chapter, several types of dermatitis have been referred, but particularly foot pad dermatitis, gangrenous dermatitis, hock burn and breast burn.

- **Dermatitis** is an inflammation of the skin. Such inflammation can be accompanied by infection, gangrene, haemorrhages and pain.
- **Gangrenous dermatitis** is characterised by a necrotization of different skin areas and a severe cellulitis of the subcutaneous tissue.
- **Pododermatitis or footpad dermatitis** is the development of lesions in the footpads of chickens, but it may occur in any part of the leg in contact with the ground. During early stages, foot rot is manifested by small erosions or discolouration of the skin.
- **Hock** (Fig. 1) **and breast burns** (Fig. 2) are marks found on the upper joints and breast of chickens raised on broiler farms. These marks are where the ammonia from the waste of other birds has burned through the skin of the leg and the breast leaving a mark.

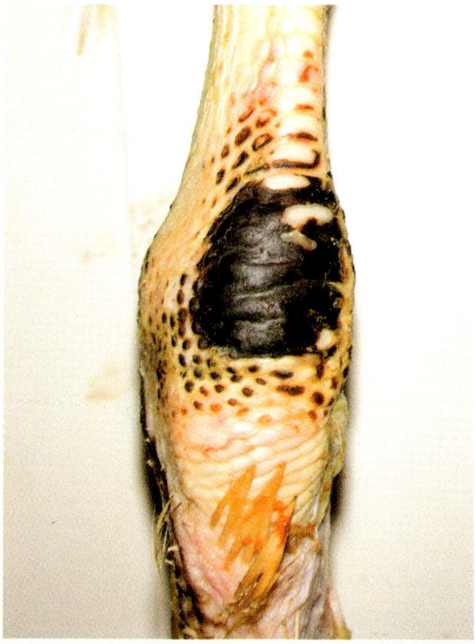

FIGURE 1. Hock burn affecting the upper joint of a broiler.

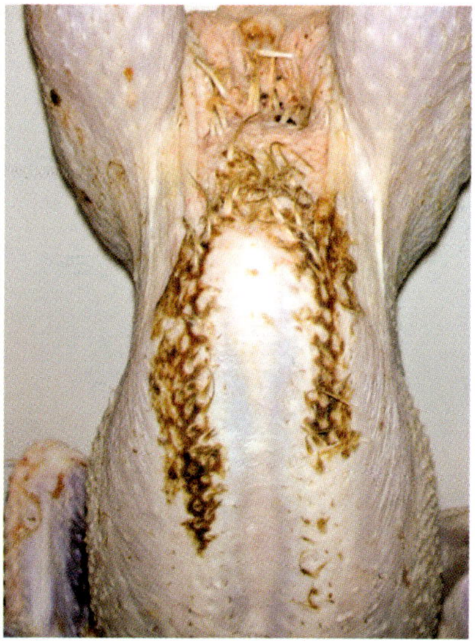

FIGURE 2. Contact dermatitis also known as breast burn produced when birds spend excessive amount of time sitting because of illness or lameness or due to inadequate bedding management.

Origin

> A poultry flock kept on well-maintained litter is healthier and more profitable than one kept on poor quality litter. Conditions such as pododermatitis, hock burn and breast blisters are, in the majority of cases, a consequence of poor litter. Secondary infections by bacteria are commonly caused by *Staphylococcus*, *Streptococcus*, *Clostridium* and erysipelas.

Gangrenous dermatitis is characterised by a necrosis of the skin, subcutaneous fluid, haemorrhages and sometimes by a cooked meat appearance of the skin (Figs. 3-6).

The origin of gangrenous dermatitis is not entirely clear, although it is thought that it begins with a scratch or aggression that becomes infected with bacteria. *Clostridium septicum, Clostridium perfringens* type A, and *Staphylococcus aureus*, either singly or in combination are most often involved.

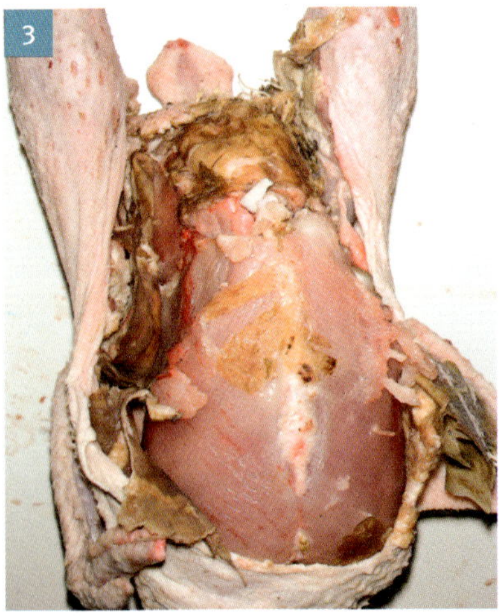

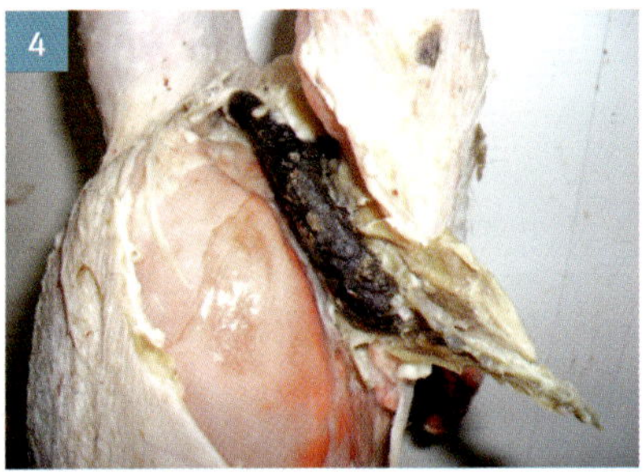

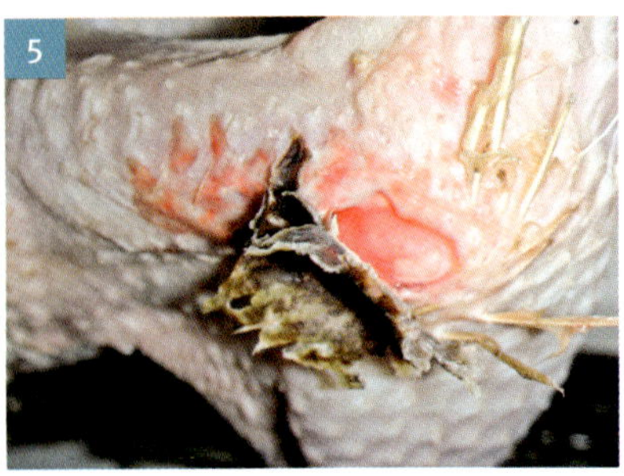

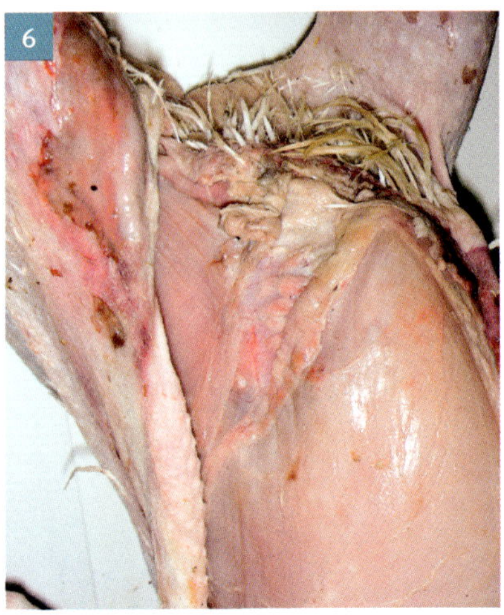

FIGURE 3. Extensive gangrenous dermatitis and severe cellulitis of the subcutaneous tissue.

FIGURE 4. Gangrenous dermatitis of the subcutaneous tissue. Petechiae and cooked meat appearance of the breast muscle.

FIGURE 5. Gangrenous dermatitis affecting a wing.

FIGURE 6. Gangrenous dermatitis to show cooked appearance of the skin.

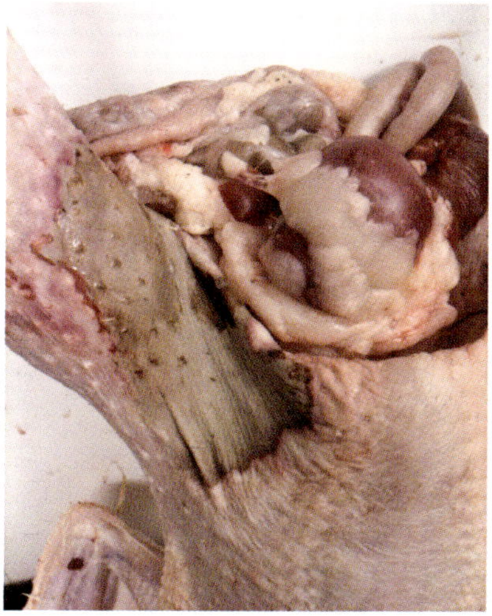

FIGURE 7. Gangrenous dermatitis of the skin. Total condemnation of the carcass is advisable.

Clostridium species are spore formers generally found in soil but can be found in feed, faeces, dust and other places. *Clostridia are* very durable and able to survive extremely harsh conditions.

Infectious diseases such as infectious bursal disease or chick anaemia virus will predispose to immune suppression and will facilitate the development of gangrenous dermatitis. Mycotoxins in the feed can also cause immune suppression. Other studies even suggest a liaison to the prevalence of coccidiosis.

Gangrenous dermatitis can become a major health problem among broiler flocks, resulting in high mortality, carcass condemnations and trimmed parts at the abattoir (Fig. 7).

Foot pad dermatitis, also known as pododermatitis or foot burn, is a condition characterised by lesions on the feet of poultry that can vary in size and also in depth. Pododermatitis is a type of contact dermatitis primarily affecting the plantar surface of the footpad often accompanied by secondary infections. The lesions are superficial in mild cases (Fig. 8) but progress into deep ulcers when the dermatitis progresses (Figs. 9 and 10), resulting in pain and discomfort to the bird. Birds with severe lesions may also show reduced weight gain duc to pain.

There are a number of predisposing factors that can influence its incidence in a flock although the biggest single factor is **wet or damp bedding**. The wetter the litter, the more likely it will promote the proliferation of pathogenic bacteria and moulds. Wet litter is also the primary cause of ammonia emissions, one of the most serious performance and environmental factors affecting broiler production today. Controlling litter moisture is the most important step in avoiding ammonia problems.

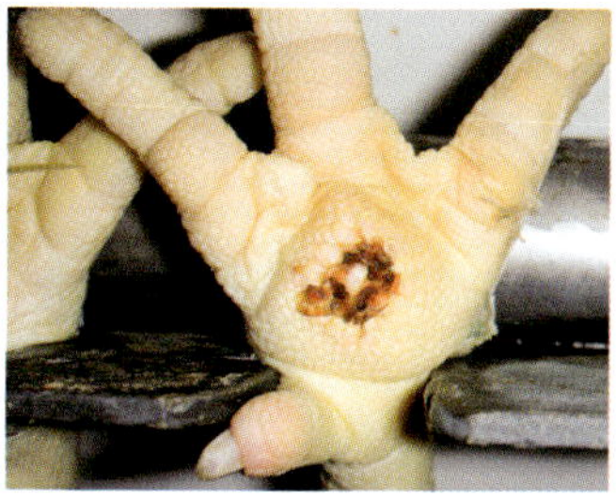

FIGURE 8. Minor lesion of the foot: mild pododermatitis.

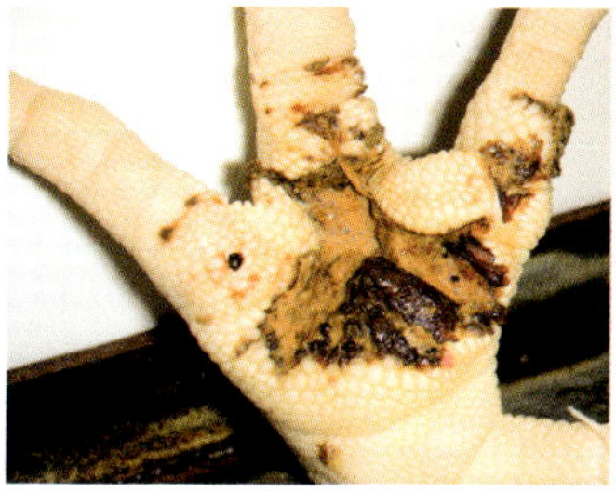

FIGURE 9. Severe pododermatitis with deep ulceration of the plantar surface of the footpad.

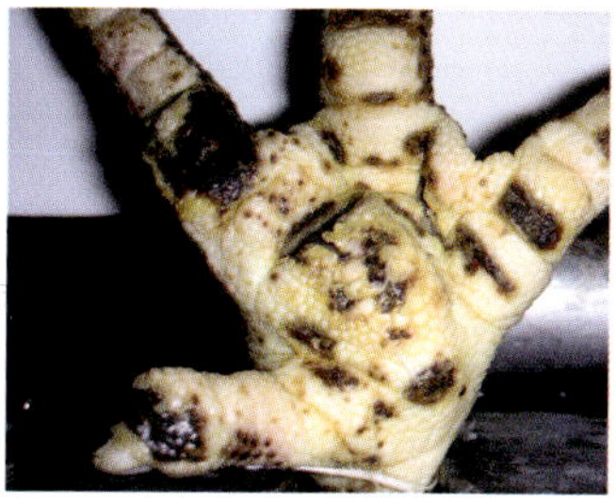

FIGURE 10. Extensive pododermatitis affecting most of the plantar surface.

Experimental evidence suggests that the worst burning tends to occur when the nitrogen content of the litter exceeds 5.5 %. The quality and amount of protein in the feed should be examined if litter nitrogen levels are high. At these times, the moisture content of the litter is also often found to be high.

There are a number of factors that influence the quality of the bed (Fig. 11):

- **Bedding material and depth**: poor quality litter will have an effect in friability and absorption capacity. There are a number of bedding materials which can be used in broiler houses. Any material in contact with the birds must be non-toxic and able to absorb water and subsequently release the moisture to the atmosphere. The material must be readily available in sufficient quantities.
- **Management of the drinking line**: this is one of the most important factors that can affect the litter quality. A poor drinker design or bad management will waste water leading to a wet litter.
- **Air change rate and house environment**: there are three different factors to be considered and these are environment temperature, humidity and ventilation. The humidity of the poultry house is affected by the number and size of birds and therefore by their respiratory output. When the relative humidity increases to an excessive level then the moisture in the litter tends to increase making the conditions poorer. When ventilation rates are not sufficient then the ammonia levels will increase and also the risk of skin burning.
- **Nutrition:** any dietary factor that causes the birds increase their water consumption is likely to lead to wetter litter. Particular attention needs to be paid to contents of sodium and chloride, potassium, crude protein, amino acids and added fat.
- **Flock health:** any disease or skeletal abnormality that decreases the birds' mobility is likely to affect their welfare adversely, as they will have increased contact with the litter. Enteritis and disorders such as the malabsorption syndrome can result in an increased excretion of water in the faeces. Likewise, Gumboro disease is well known to result in extremely wet litter.
- **Stocking density:** most of the water, fat and nitrogen found in the litter have been excreted from the birds as faeces. Therefore, the higher the density, the more of these factors the litter has to absorb. The rate of evaporation of moisture from the litter falls as stocking density increases, so particular attention must be paid to litter quality as the birds approach killing weight.

The incidence and severity of pododermatitis is of great concern to the meat industry, not only from a product quality but also from an animal welfare point of view.

FIGURE 11. Factors that can have an effect in the litter condition and consequently in the apparition of pododermatitis, hock burn and breast burn.

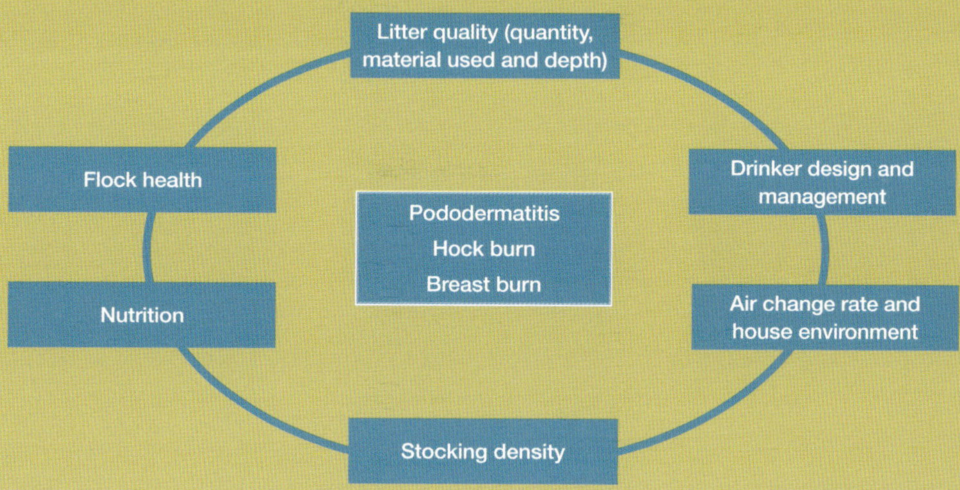

FIGURE 12. Dermatitis with cutaneous inflammatory response of the skin. Also signs of folliculitis and early stages of gangrenous dermatitis. Total rejection of the carcass and associated offal.

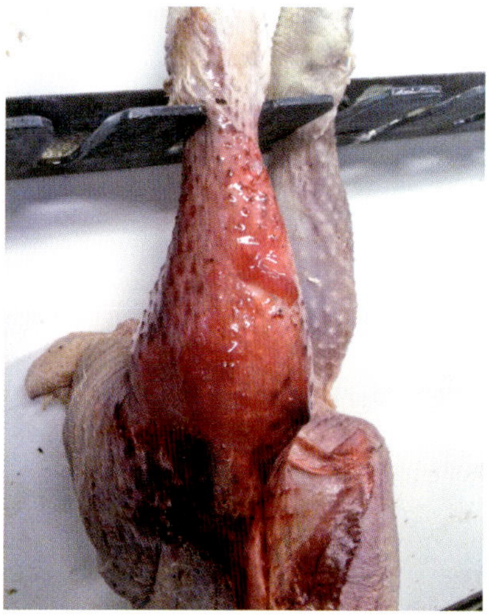

Responsibilities

Dermatitis, and in particular pododermatitis, is a multifactor problem with economic consequences. It is also an animal welfare concern which affects the walking ability of chickens reducing food intake and growth. The incidence of pododermatitis is used as objective audit criteria in welfare assessment of poultry production systems all over the world.

In general, a carcass affected by dermatitis is condemned in its entirety (Fig. 12). However, when the lesion is localised and the rest of the carcass is healthy, it may be considered removing the affected part and keeping the rest (Figs. 13-15).

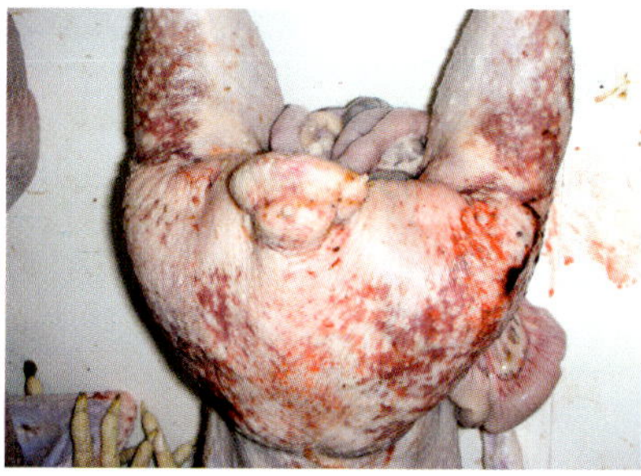

FIGURE 13. Superficial skin pigmentation. No secondary infection associated. Partial rejection is possible.

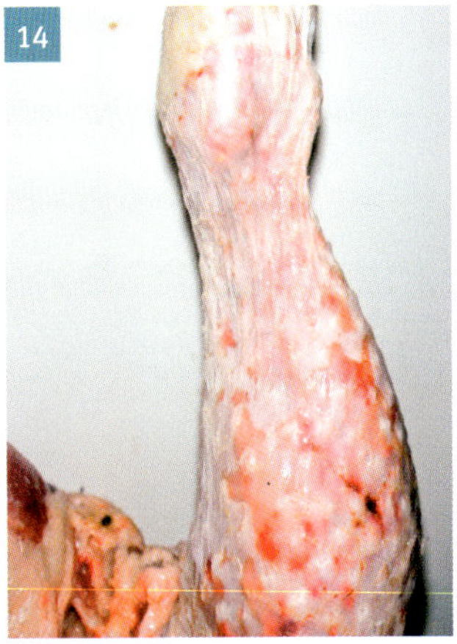

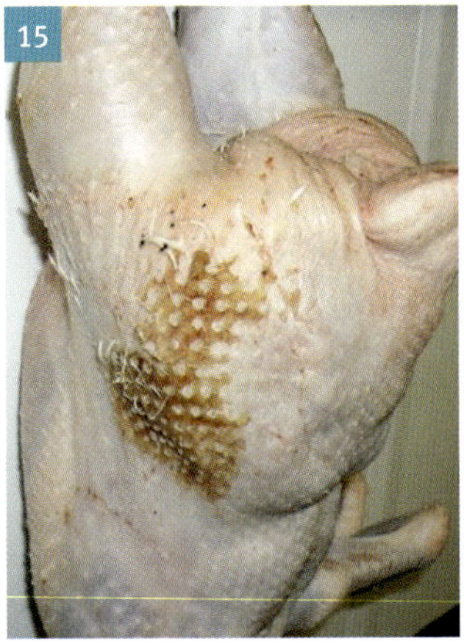

FIGURE 14. Folliculitis is an inflammation of the feather follicles. Partial rejection is possible when not associated with other lesions such cellulitis, septicaemia, emaciation or abnormal odour.

FIGURE 15. Scabby hip dermatitis characterised by dry scabs of the caudal dorsal convexity of the carcass. The aetiology is unclear and thought to be due to traumatic excoriations, resulting from birds climbing on one another at high placement densities. *Cl. perfringens* and *Staphylococcus* may colonise the skin lesions. The carcass can be trimmed when there are no signs of infection or subcutaneous cellulitis.

Severe cases of dermatitis in any of its forms need to be reported to the local authority should they need to be further investigated.

The following two pictures (Figs. 16 and 17) were taken as evidence as part of a referral for investigation in which there was a serious breach of the welfare regulations. The totality of birds were seriously affected with severe pododermatitis characterised by deep necrotic ulcers of the plantar surface of the foot pad suggesting that the flock had been maintained in extremely poor conditions during a long period of time. This incident was immediately reported to the competent authority and also discussed with the producer and the Food Business Operator.

> Remember: not all hock burn or breast blisters are simply a result of poor litter quality. If birds spend excessive amounts of time squatting down due to leg problems or other diseases they will be more likely to suffer from these lesions regardless of litter condition.

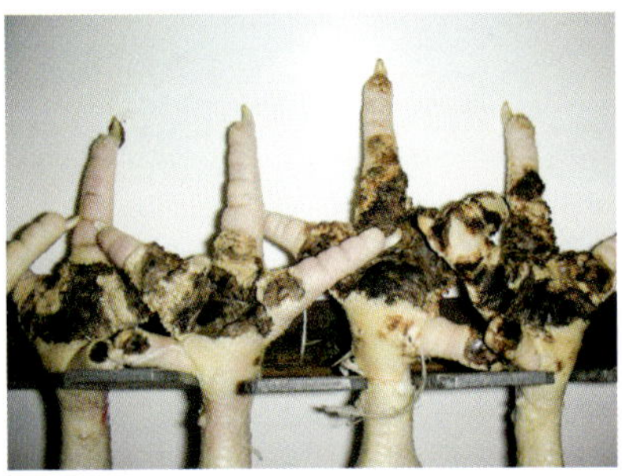

FIGURE 16. Extensive pododermatitis. Note the extension of the necrotic area of the plantar surface.

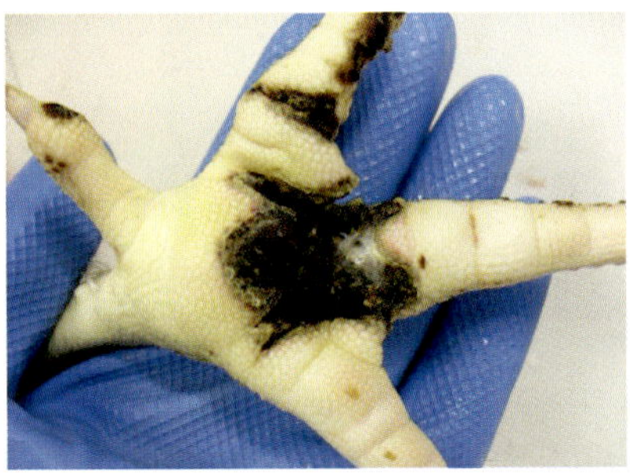

FIGURE 17. Deep ulcers are painful to the birds. The inspector and veterinarian should always report such cases as part of their routine inspection at abattoirs.

7

Airsacculitis

Definition

Birds pass air through the lungs by means of **air sacs**, a uniquely avian anatomical feature. The air sacs are balloon-like structures at the "ends" of the airway system. In the chicken there are nine such sacs: an unpaired one in the cervical region, two interclavicular air sacs, two abdominal air sacs, two anterior thoracic air sacs and two posterior thoracic air sacs. In addition, the avian respiratory system plays an important role in thermoregulation. Since birds do not have a diaphragm, they depend on the movement of the sternum (keel) and rib cage in order to breathe. Holding a bird too tight will restrict movement of the rib cage and suffocate the bird.

> Airsacculitis is defined as an inflammation of the lining of the air sacs (Fig. 1). Depending on the severity of the lesions, such inflammation will range from a slight opacity of the serosa with a small amount of watery or foamy discharge to an opaque serosa with purulent exudates (Fig. 2). Such injuries can affect one or more air sacs and sometimes be accompanied by peritonitis and pericarditis.

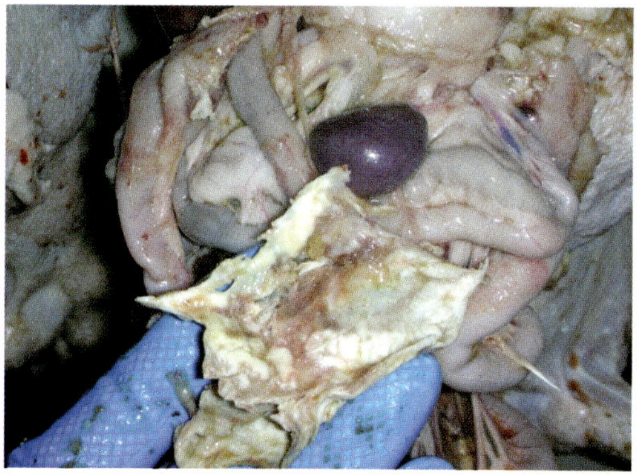

FIGURE 1. Thicker and opaque sacs.

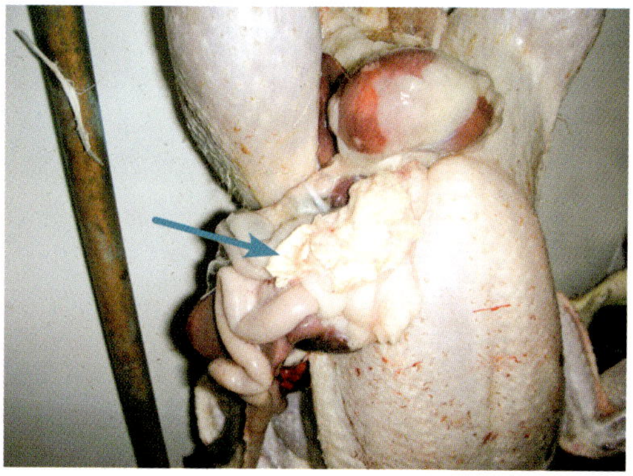

FIGURE 2. Purulent caseous airsacculitis.

Origin

The anatomy of the broiler has a huge role to play in relation to the apparition of airsacculitis. Air sacs have a very limited blood supply and nearly non-existent mechanisms of defence to fight bacteria and dust. Air sacs will get overwhelmed with dust when the conditions are not ideal and the birds are open-mouth breathing.

Respiratory diseases are grouped into either infectious or non-infectious:

- **Non-infectious causes** relate to the farm environment, particularly in relation to ventilation and the litter conditions. To this extent, ammonia and dust levels play an important role in the apparition of airsacculitis. Ammonia is produced by the degradation of the faeces and its levels are directly related to other factors such as temperature in the house, pH of the litter, ventilation and aeration. A poorly ventilated and dusty environment is the most significant factor associated with respiratory disease and consequently with high level of rejection during processing. It is thought that inhalation of dust contaminated with faeces is the cause of secondary *E. coli* airsacculitis.
- **Infectious causes** could be of bacterial, viral, mycoplasmal or fungal aetiology.

Responsibilities

Airsacculitis represents a cost to producers and growers, mortality at the farms, therapeutic costs and excess condemnations. The data collected at post-mortem inspection is used as an indication of the health status of the flock, assisting veterinarians in the investigation of the source of the problem.

The main responsibility will be to detect the condition and to take a decision on the wholesomeness of the carcass. Carcasses and associated offal affected by airsacculitis are generally condemned (Figs. 3 and 4), particularly if accompanied by perihepatitis, pericarditis or peritonitis (Fig. 5).

Some establishments may have a system in place to salvage carcasses when the affected parts can be removed safely and in a hygienic manner. There are nine air sacs in the chicken: unpaired clavicular and paired cervical, cranial thoracic, caudal thoracic and abdominal air sacs. The cervical and interclavicular air sacs connect to bone and the anterior deep pectoral muscle. Such a complex respiratory system makes salvage of the affected carcasses a challenge for any company hence they are normally condemned by the inspector or veterinarian. Total condemnation is, in most cases, the most appropriate decision (Fig. 6).

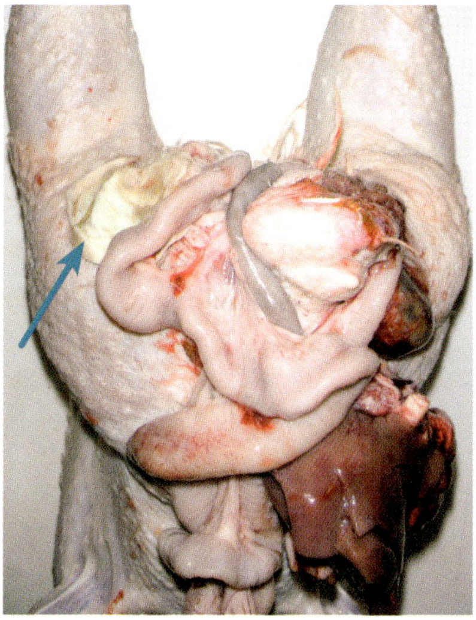

FIGURE 3. Airsacculitis affecting a single air sac. Condemnation of viscera only.

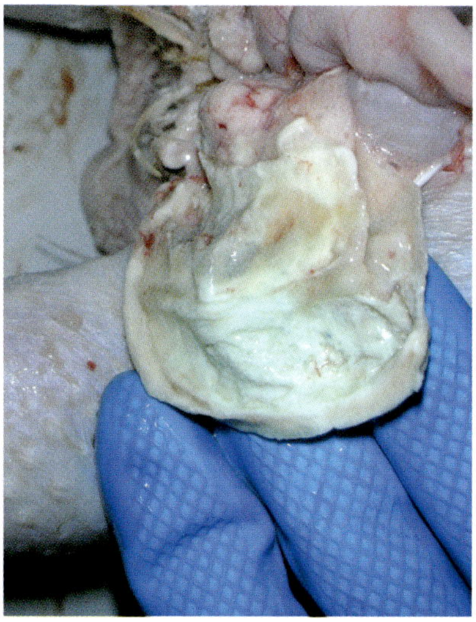

FIGURE 4. Airsacculitis affecting a single air sac. Rejection of the viscera.

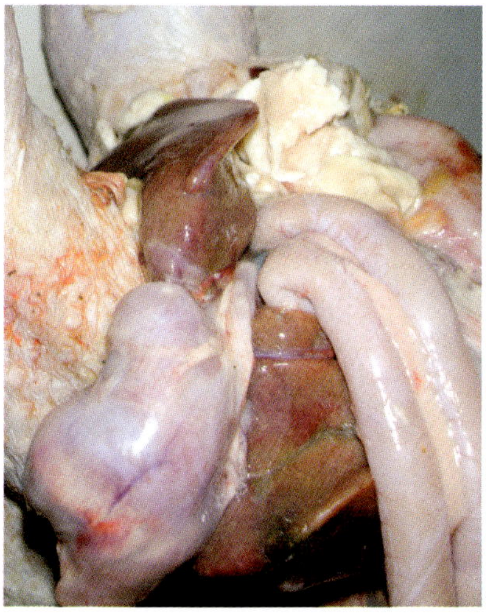

FIGURE 5. Airsacculitis and pericarditis associated with hepatitis. Total condemnation of the carcass and viscera.

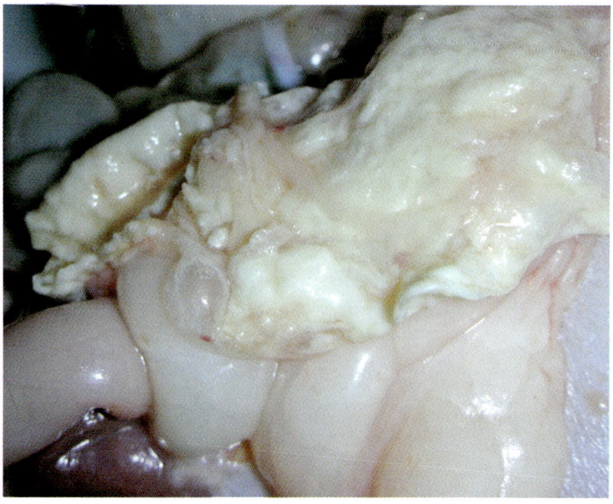

FIGURE 6. Chronic purulent airsacculitis. Total condemnation of the carcass.

The following pictures (Fig. 7) illustrate a case of airsacculitis affecting a batch of broilers aged 52 days for which swabs were collected from the air sacs. The carcasses were all rejected as unfit for human consumption. The swabs revealed significant bacterial growth mainly *E. coli*. The bacteria could have been primary in origin or secondary to respiratory viruses such as infectious bronchitis.

Growth on Blood Agar and on Mac Agar revealed presence of *E. coli* affecting four different air sacs. Antibiogram results showed sensitivity to enrofloxacin, apramycin and colistine. The bacterium was resistant to amoxicillin, lincomycin, trimethoprim-sulfadiazine, tilosin and tiamulin.

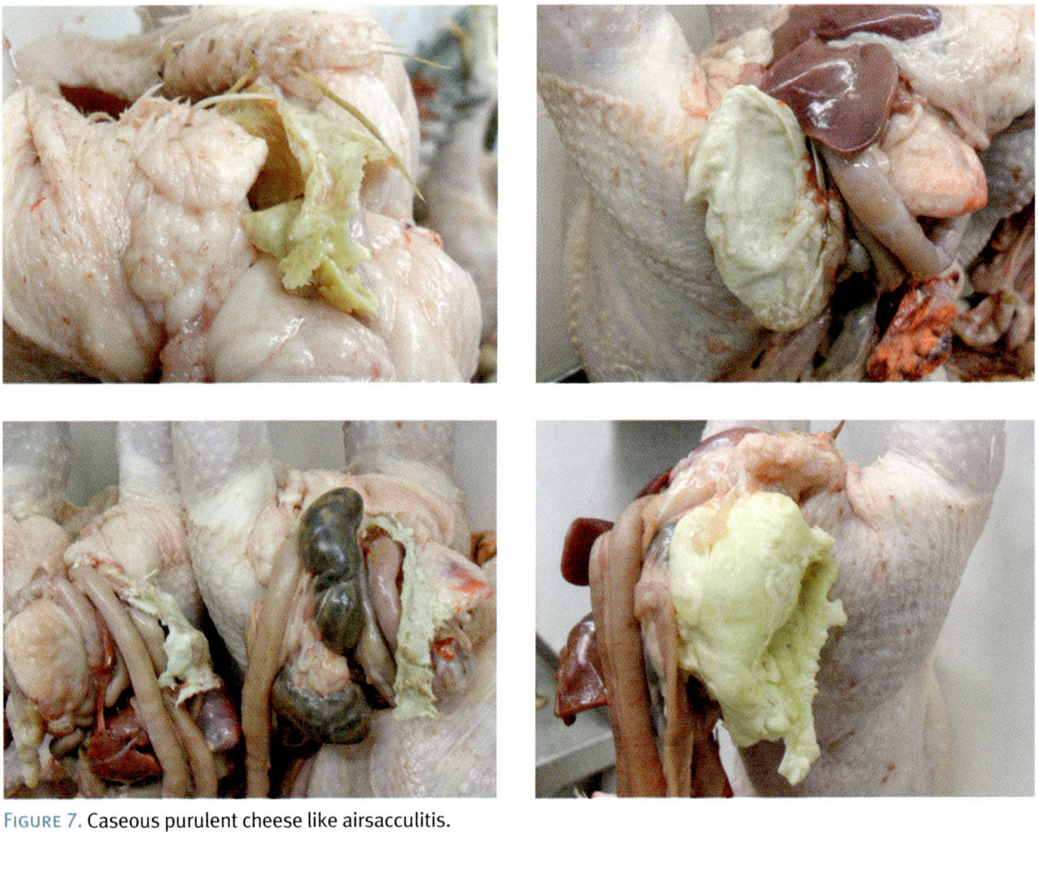

FIGURE 7. Caseous purulent cheese like airsacculitis.

8

Pericarditis

Definition

Pericarditis is an inflammatory process of the pericardium. Pericarditis also implies the accumulation of fluid between the heart and the pericardium which can lead to **hydropericardium** when excessive fluid accumulates in the pericardial cavity (Figs. 1 and 2).

Pericarditis can be found in different forms depending on the severity of the infection and the causative agent (Figs. 3 and 4). Lesions may vary from a cloudy pericardium, to adhesions of the epicardium and pericardium, to a purulent and fibrinous inflammatory process of the pericardium and/or the epicardium (Fig. 5).

1
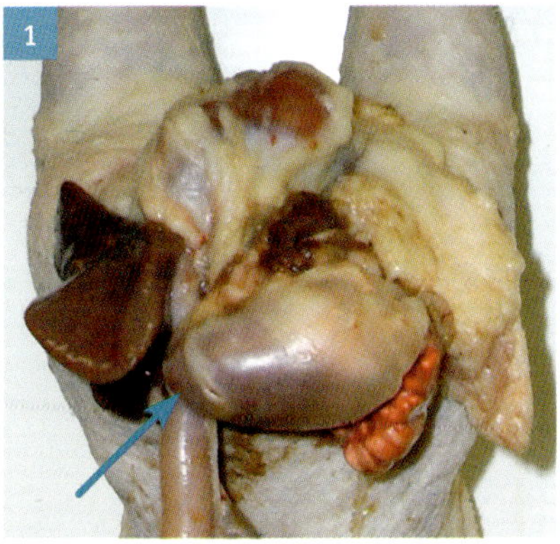

2
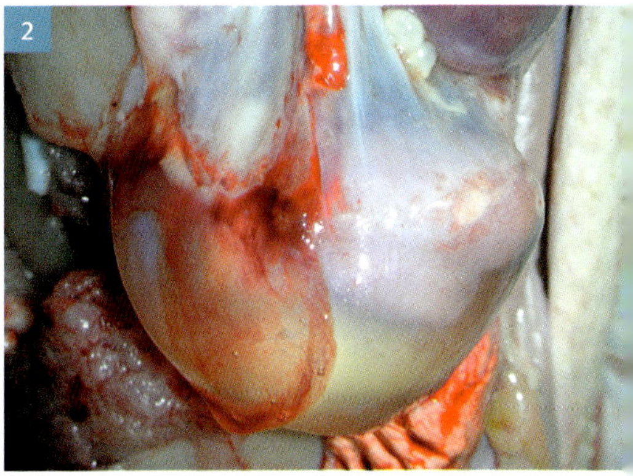

3
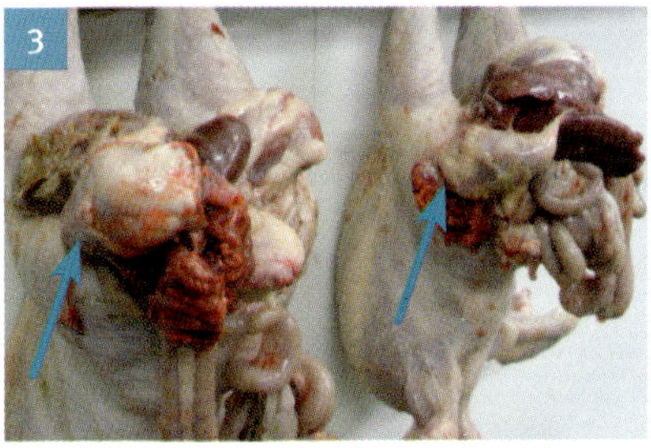

4
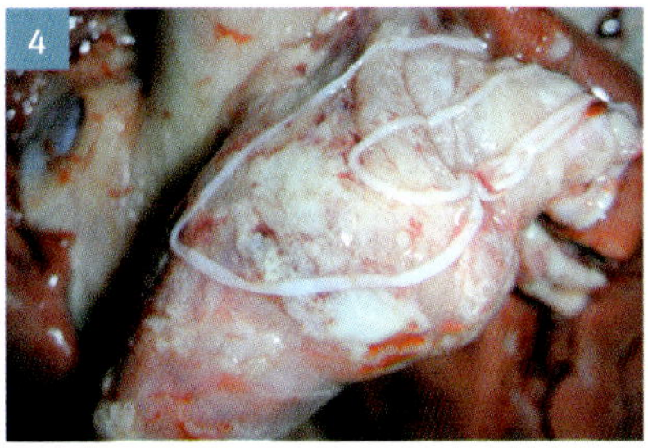

5
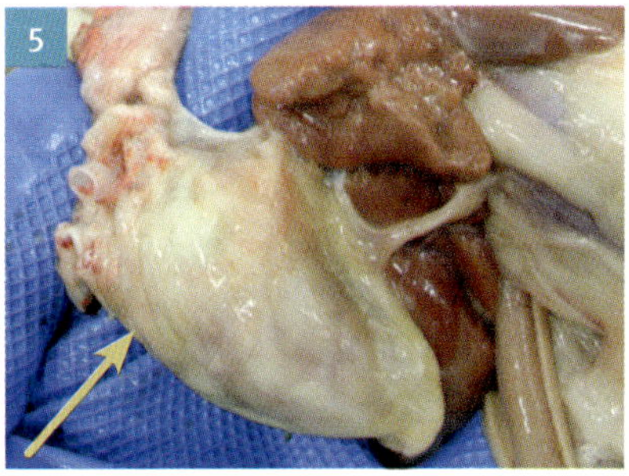

FIGURE 1. Hydropericardium with no associated conditions. Carcass passed as fit for human consumption.

FIGURE 2. Hydropericardium to show excessive amount of pericardial fluid accumulated in the pericardial space.

FIGURE 3. Severe active pericarditis affecting a flock of broilers.

FIGURE 4. Pericarditis with no other associated conditions resulting in sole rejection of the affected part.

FIGURE 5. Serofibrinous pericarditis with no other associated lesions. Offal rejected as unfit for human consumption.

Origin

Presence of pericarditis does not always mean that there is a systemic disease. Pericarditis in broilers may originate from a number of different aetiologies (Fig. 6).

FIGURE 6. **Most common causative agents in relation to the presence of pericarditis.**

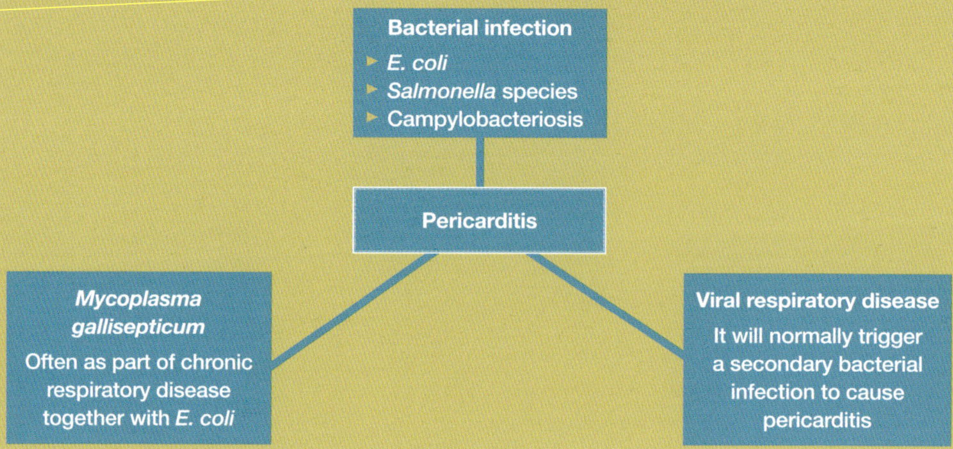

Most commonly found to be of a **bacterial infection origin**, ***E. coli*** and ***Salmonella*** frequently being isolated. *Salmonella enteritidis* will normally result in a mucopurulent pericarditis. **Campylobacteriosis** may also induce the apparition of pericarditis normally causing an adhesion of the pericardium to the surface of the heart.

Viral infections can also produce pericarditis although it is more often found in conjunction with bacteraemia or septicaemia.

Pericarditis can also be found together with **chronic respiratory disease**, which is commonly produced by *E. coli* and ***Mycoplasma gallicepticum***.

It is frequently seen that pericarditis is not found as an isolated lesion, and in many cases it have been found grouped together with perihepatitis (Figs. 7-11), peritonitis (Fig. 12) and airsacculitis. It is not uncommon to see a high incidence of pericarditis within the same batch of birds while carrying out post-mortem inspection.

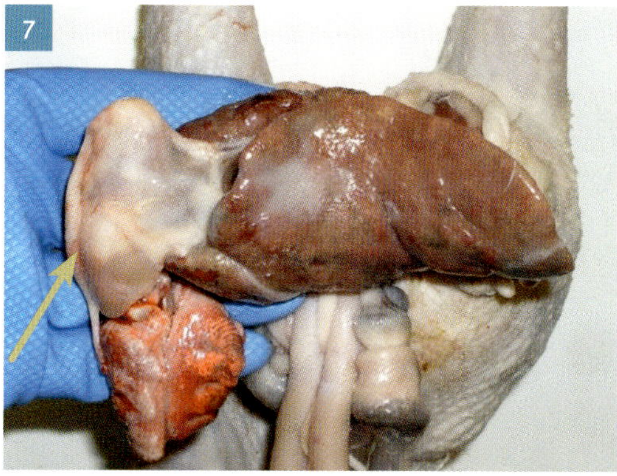

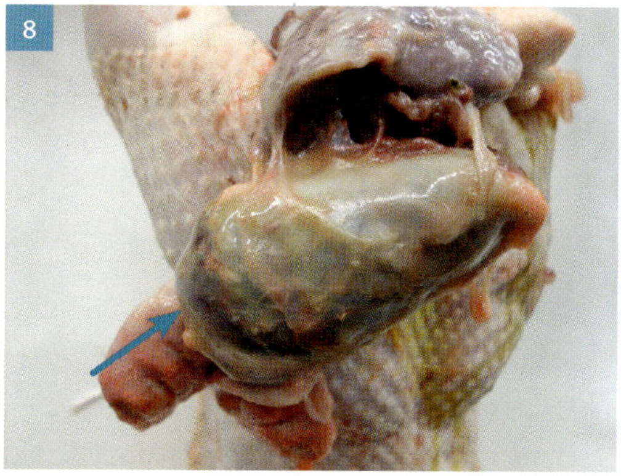

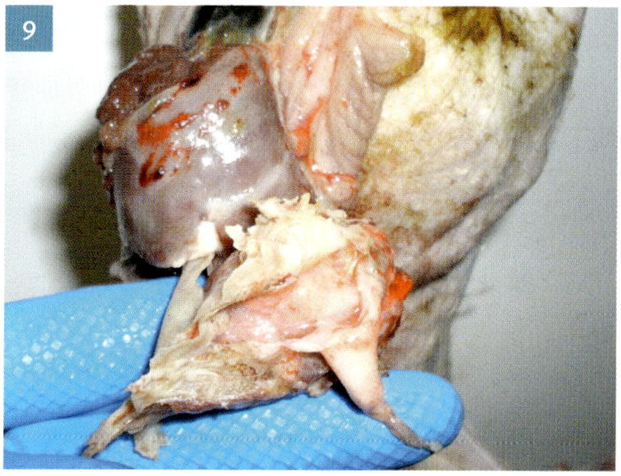

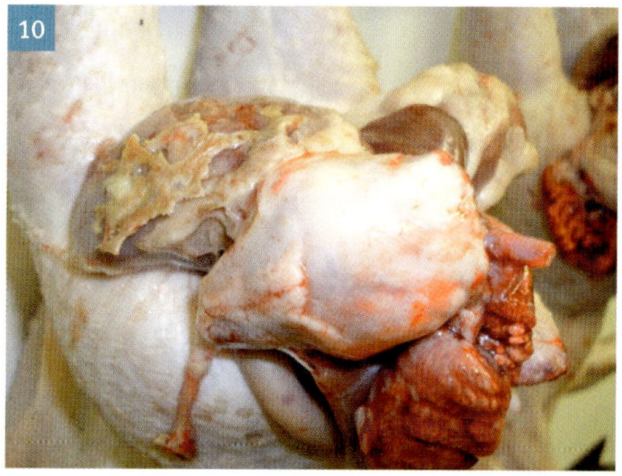

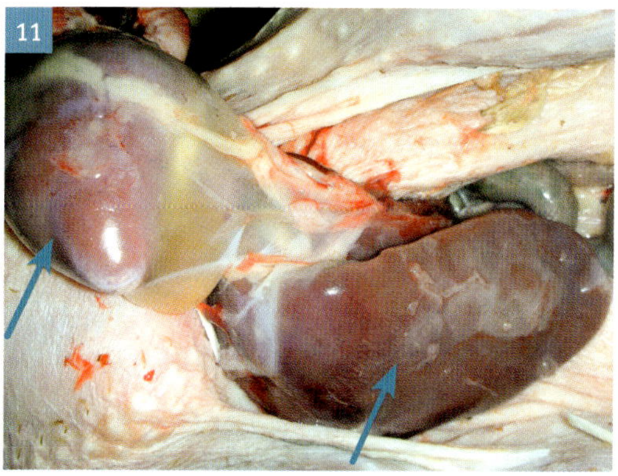

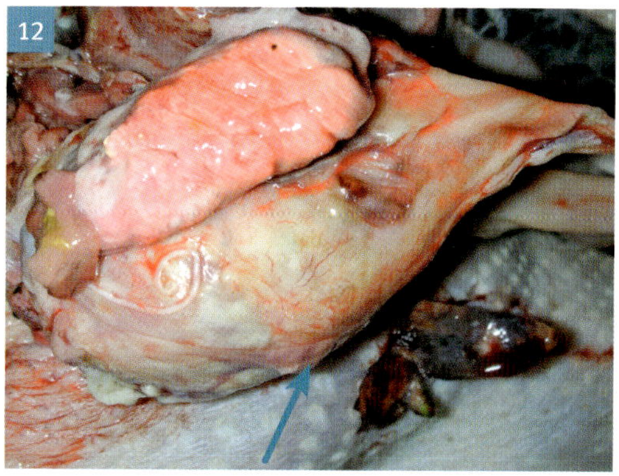

FIGURE 7. Severe active pericarditis with associated hepatitis. Total rejection of the carcass and offal.

FIGURE 8. Severe purulent pericarditis and perihepatitis rendering carcass and associated offal unfit for human consumption.

FIGURE 9. Active purulent pericarditis and associated perihepatitis. Total rejection of the carcass and offal.

FIGURE 10. Pericarditis and perihepatitis showing severe inflammatory response with purulent tissue surrounding the heart and liver.

FIGURE 11. Hydropericardium associated with perihepatitis. Carcass and offal are unfit for human consumption.

FIGURE 12. Chronic pericarditis. Note the thickness of the white inflammatory tissue that surrounds the heart. This carcass was also affected with a severe peritonitis rendering both the carcass and the offal as unfit for human consumption.

Responsibilities

The outcome of the inspection relies on a judgement made by the inspector. As previously mentioned, the presence of pericarditis does not mean that there is a general infection, so the inspector should take into consideration the general condition of the carcass and other associated conditions if any. Severely affected batches may require the speed of the line to be reduced so as to ensure a more detailed post-mortem inspection. European law currently requires testing for *Salmonella* in farms prior to slaughter. The inspector will need to take into account the outcome of such results in assessing the wholesomeness of the carcass. ***Salmonella enteritidis*** and ***Salmonella typhimurium*** have accounted for the majority of cases of human salmonellosis since the 1980s and have consistently been the most commonly implicated pathogens in general outbreaks of foodborne disease. Statutory requirements for the monitoring and control of *Salmonella* contained in EU Regulations (EC) No 2160/2003 and (EC) No 646/2007 are intended to ensure that, for the protection of human health, coherent action to reduce *Salmonella* serotypes considered to be of particular human health significance (*S. enteritidis* and *typhimurium*) is taken across the Community.

Always refer to the latest legislation in force with regards to *Salmonella* testing requirements since this may have an influence in post-mortem inspection judgements.

9

Emaciation

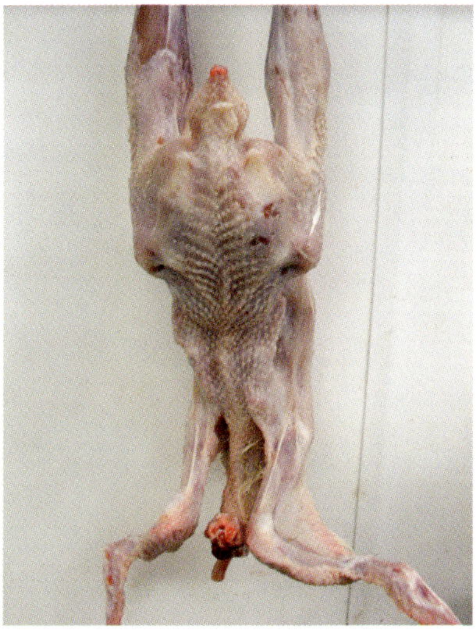

FIGURE 1. Dorsal view of an emaciated carcass. This carcass was also showing signs of dehydration and septicaemia.

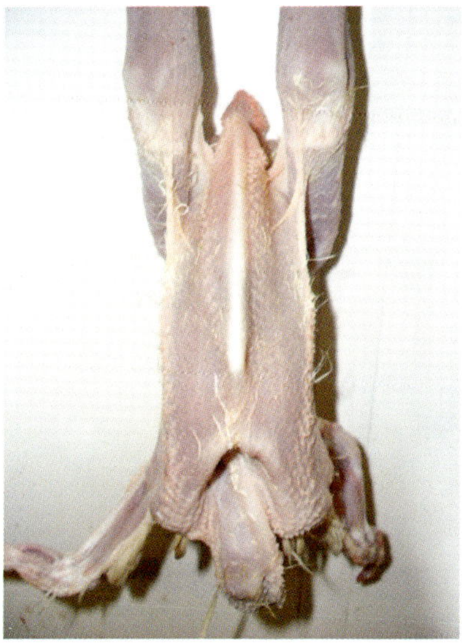

FIGURE 2. Emaciated carcass unfit for human consumption. Note palpable sternum indicating under development of the breast muscles.

Definition

Emaciation is a condition relatively frequent during broiler inspection. It is characterised by a loss of substantial amounts of fat and muscles, making the carcass look extremely thin. Emaciation is commonly accompanied by other conditions such as septicaemia and dehydration (Fig. 1).

> It is important to differentiate emaciated birds from small but well fleshed ones which, unless affected by other conditions, should not be condemned.

Affected carcasses are smaller than the rest of the same flock and show under developed muscles, particularly the breast muscles. A good indication of emaciation is the presence of a distinguishable and palpable sternum (Fig. 2).

Emaciated birds or high mortality have been used by veterinarians and farmers effectively for many years in the evaluation of the health and welfare of on-farm broiler flocks.

Origin

Emaciation in broilers is caused due to a malnutrition process in which there is a limitation in the access of food. Genetic diversity may condition the size of some chickens, limiting their access to reach food and being unable to compete with the rest of the group. Other origins of emaciation include partial paralysis, for example in the case of spondylolisthesis.

> Poor management at the farm of origin may exacerbate the problem, particularly when associated with inadequate density of birds in the sheds, poor ventilation or inadequate bedding.

Cachexia is a similar condition to emaciation but is due to a pathological condition: either a bacterial or a viral infection.

Neither of these conditions is differentiated at post-mortem inspection and they are treated equally, normally as emaciated carcasses. The cause of the condition cannot be determined during the inspection and either way these carcasses are rejected as unfit for human consumption.

Responsibilities

Birds suffering from emaciation or caquexia should not reach the slaughterhouse in the first place and they should be slaughtered at the farm when the condition is first detected. Some of these birds are inevitably undetected during the catching process and they reach the slaughterhouse where there are certain animal welfare implications to be considered (Fig. 3). First of all, smaller birds are more likely to miss the stunner and the automatic neck cutter (when used) and consequently they are at risk of not being stunned and bled at all. The inspector or veterinarian should always consider this possibility in order to reassure the welfare of those birds.

A high incidence of emaciation implies a pathological problem or a management problem at the farm and this should be considered by the inspector in suspecting a potential breach of the animal welfare regulations. Competent authorities must be informed accordingly.

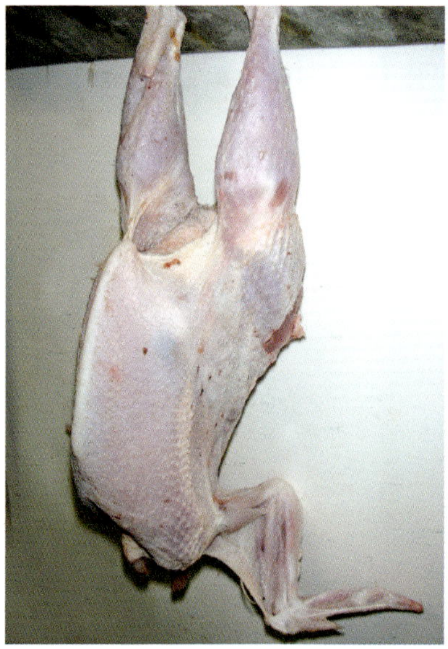

FIGURE 3. Emaciated carcass. Poor development of the breast muscles. Total rejection of the carcass.

It is important to differentiate small but well fleshed chickens from emaciated carcasses which should be with no exemption declared as unfit for human consumption. Small birds with no signs of malnutrition should be passed as fit for human consumption.

10

Hepatitis

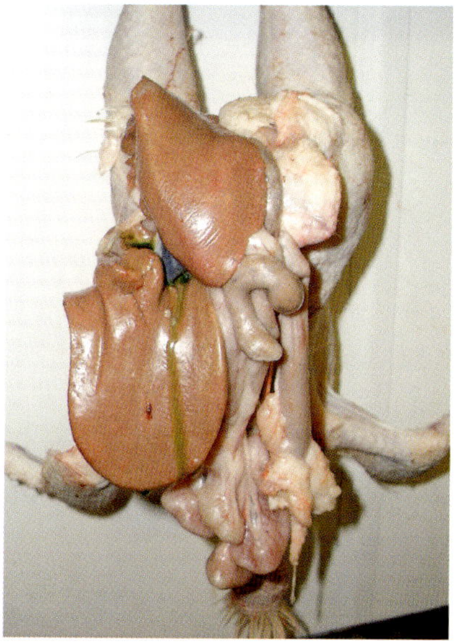

FIGURE 1. Cholangiohepatitis. Note enlarged liver with a firm, smooth surface and discolouration. This carcass was passed as fit for human consumption with no other conditions detected. Associated offal was discarded.

Definition

Affection or inflammatory disease of the liver: frequently found during day-to-day post-mortem inspection, this condition is the most common cause of partial rejection. Hepatitis can be present in different forms although this chapter will refer to the most frequent ones:

- **Hepatosis or cholangiohepatitis** (Fig. 1): inflammatory and dystrophic process of the bile ducts and the liver parenchyma. The liver appears enlarged with rounded edges and a paler colour. Sometimes mottled with multiple small greyish-white or greenish foci.
- **Focal liver necrosis:** multiple localised necrosis of the liver parenchyma and inflammatory process of the liver as a response to such necrosis and its causative agent.
- **Jaundice:** also known as icterus, it is characterised in broiler inspection by a yellowish pigmentation of the carcass and associated offal.

Origin

Hepatosis or cholangiohepatitis has its origin in the migration of bacteria, viruses or toxins from the intestine into the bile ducts. The resulting inflammation of the intrahepatic bile ducts alters the normal flow of bile which leaches back into the hepatic parenchyma. The liver appears enlarged with a paler yellow colour and its surface feels firm (Fig. 2). Size and colour may vary enormously.

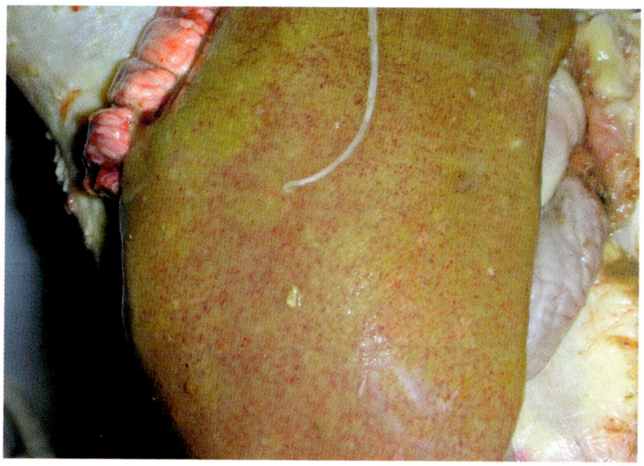

FIGURE 2. Enlarged liver with cholangiohepatitis. Note inflammation of the parenchyma with a yellowish discolouration of the liver.

In some cases, its surface has a characteristic acinous appearance and in others is mottled with multiple small greyish-white or greenish foci. The gallbladder's walls can in some cases appear thickened and opaque, and it is often found associated cholecystitis and extra hepatic bile ducts distended with bile.

Histopathologically, there is fibrosis with proliferation of biliary ductules, cholestasis and heterophilic and lymphocytic infiltration.

The development of this liver condition is not one hundred per cent understood, and although *Cl. perfringens* has been suggested as the most common causative agent, the precise pathogenesis of the hepatic lesions remains unclear.

Bacteria and toxins could potentially be transported in the blood through damaged gut mucosa from the intestines to the liver. In fact, cholangiohepatitis has been observed in conjunction with necrotic enteritis and several studies suggest a relation between the two conditions. *Cl. perfringens* can produce a significant amount of toxins which can eventually induce gut tissue necrosis. Both bacteria and toxins could be transported through a damaged mucosa to the liver by the blood. Another possibility is an ascending infection via the bile tree which could eventually trigger an inflammatory process of the bile ducts and consequently an obstruction of the bile flow.

Focal hepatic necrosis (Fig. 3) is commonly found at post-mortem inspection and it is characterised by localised necrosis of the liver surface and parenchyma. Different bacterial strains have been isolated such as *E. coli*, *S. aureus*, *Cl. perfringens* and Streptococcus, and also certain toxins. There is no standard

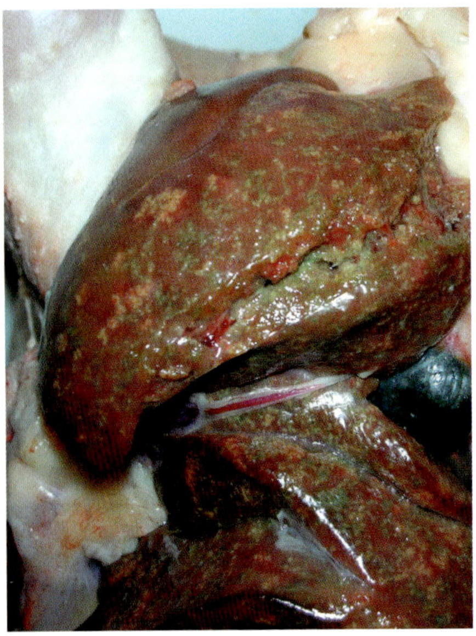

FIGURE 3. Focal necrosis of the liver. Offal should be rejected.

pattern as far as lesions are concerned; there is a huge variation in colour, size and shape of these multifocal necrotic-like livers, from pale or whitish with hepatic granulomas to green with multifocal necrosis.

There seems to be a relation between intestinal health balance and focal hepatic necrosis or bacterial necrosis. Duodenal microbiota can be altered during rearing by many factors, such as stress, antibiotic treatments, a virus infection, the use of growth promoters, etc., which could lead to an opportunistic bacterial infection. Such infection is characterised by the proliferation of bacterial species that are not naturally present in that region. It makes sense to think that bacteria and toxins could then be transported to the liver via the portal circulatory system to induce hepatocite necrosis.

Livers affected by hepatitis are not normally isolated cases within a batch of birds, so the inspector should expect a high incidence of them at times while undertaking inspection duties.

Jaundice (Figs. 4-6) is the result of a hyperbilirubinaemia or increased level of bilirubin in the blood. Author's practical experience tells that jaundice in broilers is more commonly found following a liver disease. Hepatocite necrosis reduces the liver's ability to metabolise and excrete bilirubin leading to a build-up of unconjugated bilirubin in the blood. There is a post-hepatic icterus also known as obstructive in which the flow of bile into the duodenum is disrupted due to cholangitis or enteritis.

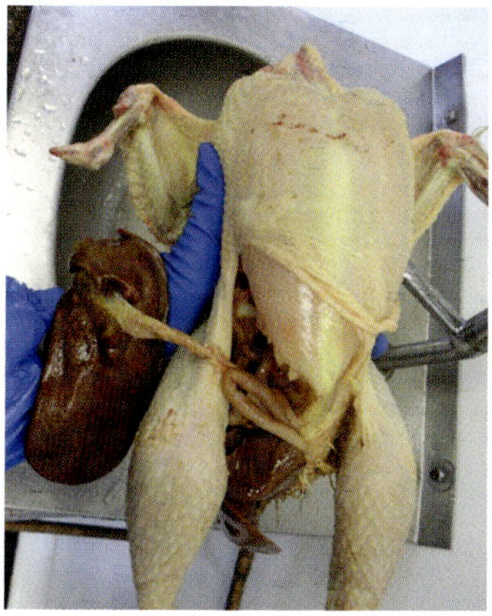

FIGURE 4. A jaundice carcass. Enlarged liver and discolouration.

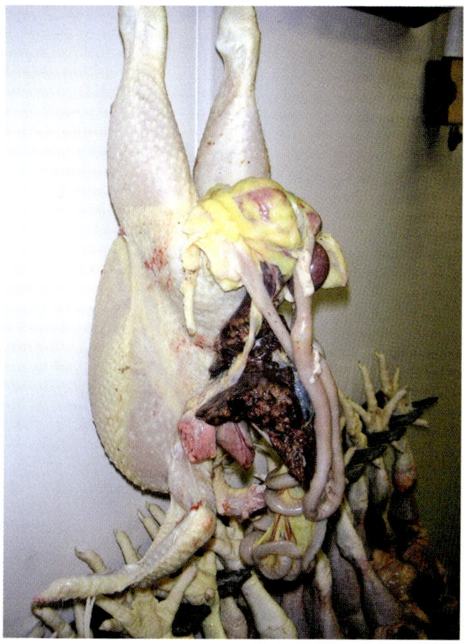

FIGURE 5. Acute jaundice affecting a broiler carcass. Note yellowish tinge of the surrounding fat and skin due to the deposition of bile pigments. All carcasses and associated offal should be rejected.

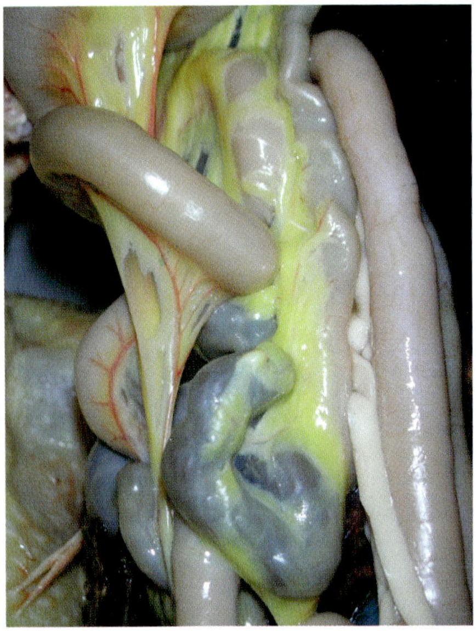

FIGURE 6. Yellowish tinge of the intestinal fat in a jaundice bird. There is deposition of bile pigments in the fat and other tissues due to an increased level of bilirubin in the blood. Such carcasses and associated offal must be rejected and they are unfit for human consumption.

Responsibilities

Hepatitis is the most common reason for partial condemnation in broilers (Fig. 7).

The inspector will need to judge the carcass upon associated lesions, if any, signs of systemic disease and general condition (Figs. 8 and 9). It is not uncommon to find hepatitis associated with pericarditis (Fig. 10). In which case, a whole bird condemnation would be required. Any signs of septicaemia, emaciation, dermatitis, airsacculitis, peritonitis or celullitis would also imply a whole carcass rejection (Fig. 11).

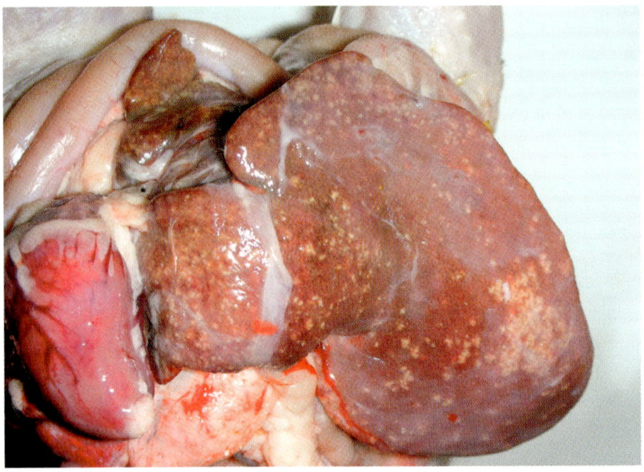

FIGURE 7. Focal hepatic necrosis with no other associated lesions. Offal must be rejected and the rest of the carcass passed as fit for human consumption.

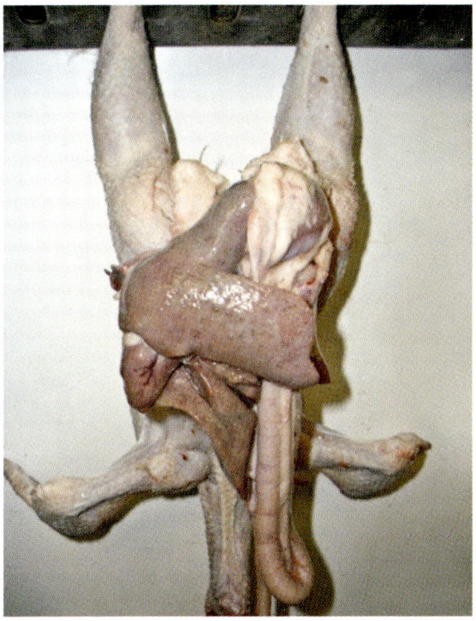

FIGURE 8. Hepatitis with no other associated disturbance. The carcass can be passed as fit for human consumption. Note enlarged liver but good general condition of the carcass.

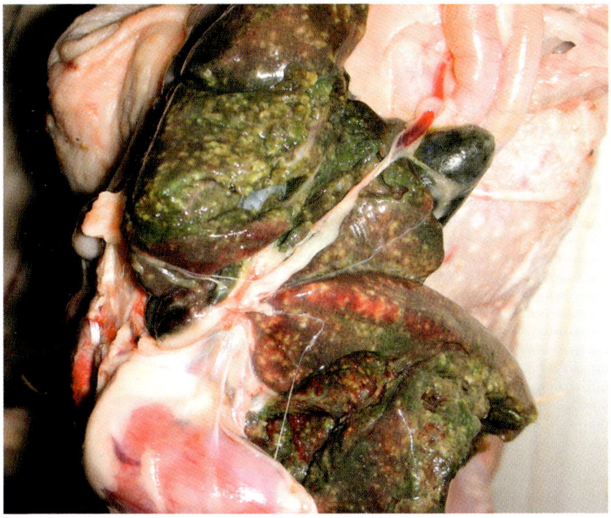

FIGURE 9. Advanced necrosis of the liver. Greenish discolouration. due to disruption of the biliary system and affection of the liver substance.

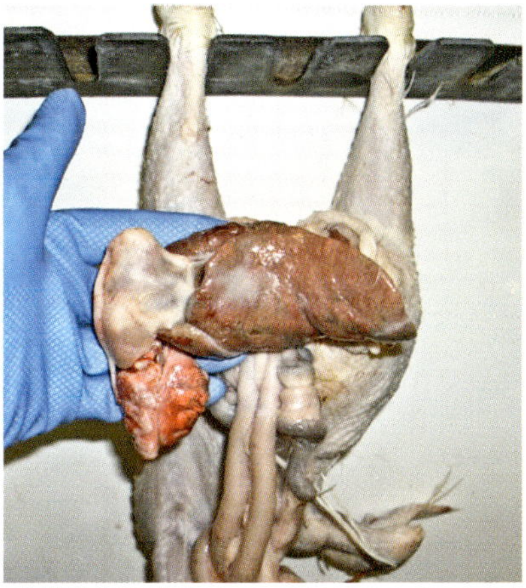

FIGURE 10. Focal hepatic necrosis associated with acute pericarditis. Whole bird rejection is applicable in such case scenario.

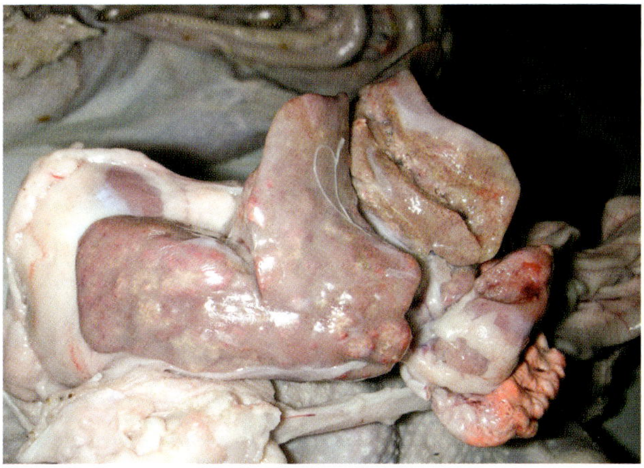

FIGURE 11. Severe hepatitis with focal hepatic necrosis. Note extensive hepatic necrosis in the form of granulomas affecting the whole liver. This carcass and associated offal were condemned based on the severity of the lesions.

It has been detected, on numerous occasions, batches severely affected with hepatitis which have had a low percentage of whole bird condemnation, and vice versa. When discarding a diseased liver, it is being aimed for the entirety of the offal within that same carcass.

> When processing a batch severely affected by hepatitis there are other considerations to be taken with regards to line speed and concentration breaks while carrying out post-mortem inspection. It is paramount in such case scenarios to make sure that partial rejection of the offal is under control to ensure that no affected livers enter the food chain. To this extent, the Food Business Operator should have a contingency plan in place in which the speed of the line can be reduced if needed. The inspection team must be confident during the whole process to guarantee that partial rejection is carried out accordingly.

It is important not to confuse a **corn fed chicken** with chickens suffering from jaundice, particularly when processing free range chickens. Look for any signs of hepatitis and enteritis, keeping in mind that jaundice cases are relatively rare (Fig. 12).

> It is important to keep records of the percentage of rejected livers in a given batch; this is valuable information to producers and veterinarians. Feedback will then be used to assess the health status of the flock and to reveal breaches in biosecurity and management at the farm, if any.

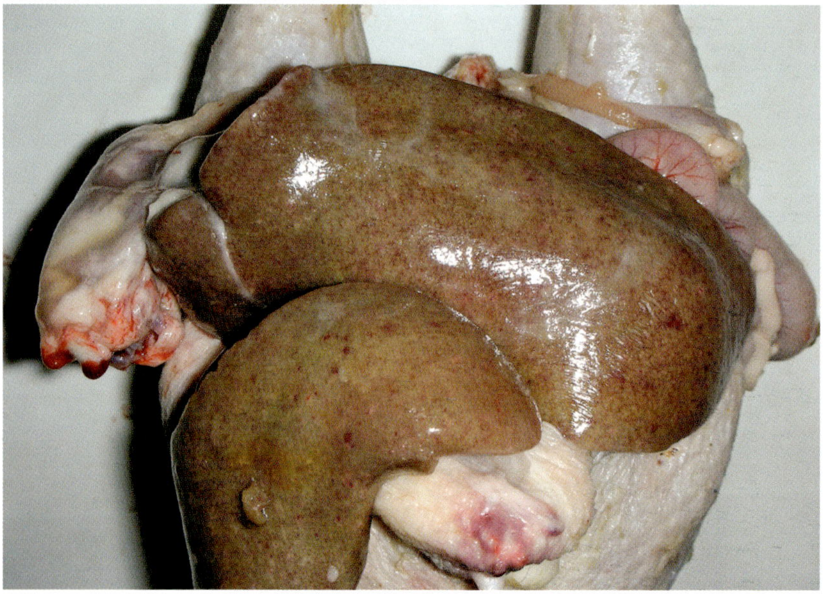

FIGURE 12. Cholangiohepatitis in a bird mildly affected with jaundice.

11

Peritonitis and perihepatitis

Definition

The peritoneum is a serous membrane that lines the walls of the pelvic abdominal cavity. This strong, colourless membrane with a smooth surface forms a double layer bag. The space between the parietal and visceral peritoneum is called the peritoneal cavity. This cavity contains, among others, the larger air sacs, most of the organs of the digestive tract (proventriculus, gizzard, small and large intestines, liver and pancreas), the genitourinary system (kidneys, ureters and ovary) and the spleen.

- **Peritonitis** is an inflammation of the peritoneum. The condition is characterised by dry caseous or mucopurulent yellow exudates in the peritoneal membrane and into any of the organs in the peritoneal cavity (Figs. 1 and 2).

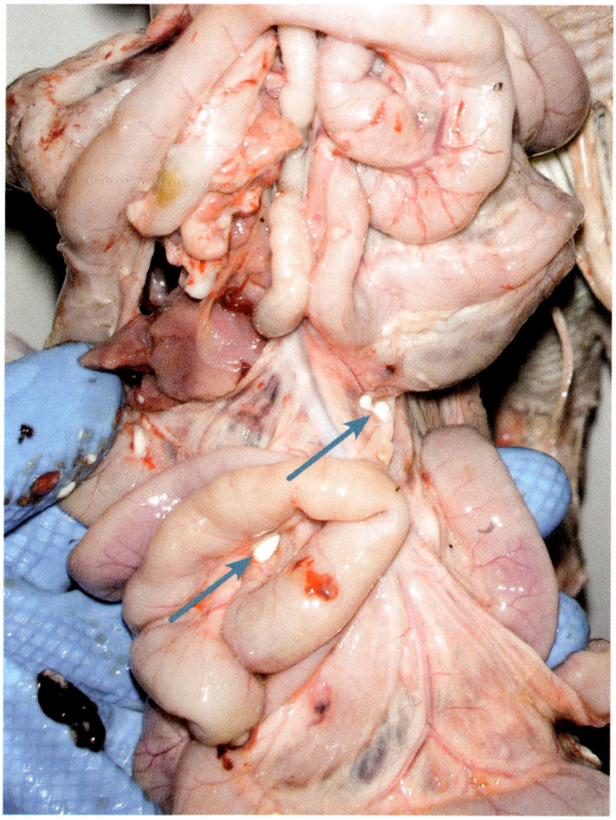

FIGURE 1. Peritonitis in the form of purulent caseous exudates in the abdominal cavity in between the intestines. This form of peritonitis can be difficult to detect when there are no other associated conditions. Carcass and offal are unfit for human consumption and they are rejected accordingly.

- **Perihepatitis** can be described as a type of visceral peritonitis characterised by an inflammation of the peritoneal coating of the liver. Lesions vary from slight adherent fibrous attachments to large and thickened fibrous attachments to the outside surface of the liver (Figs. 3-5).

Both conditions can be relatively common at post-mortem inspection point.

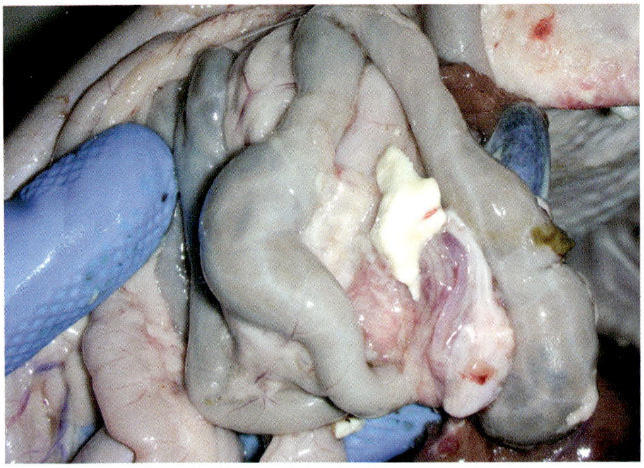

FIGURE 2. Caseous exudates indicating peritonitis.

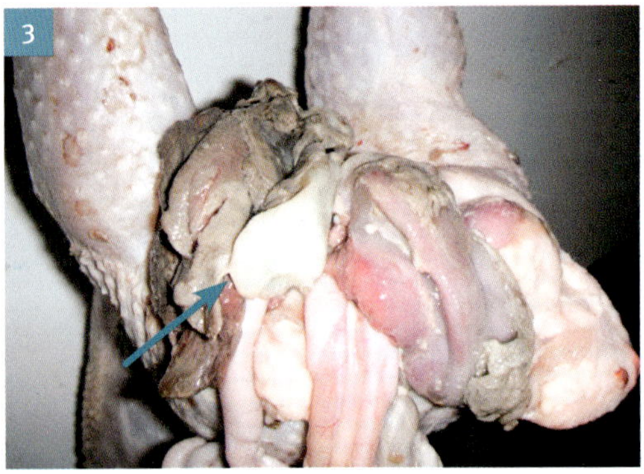

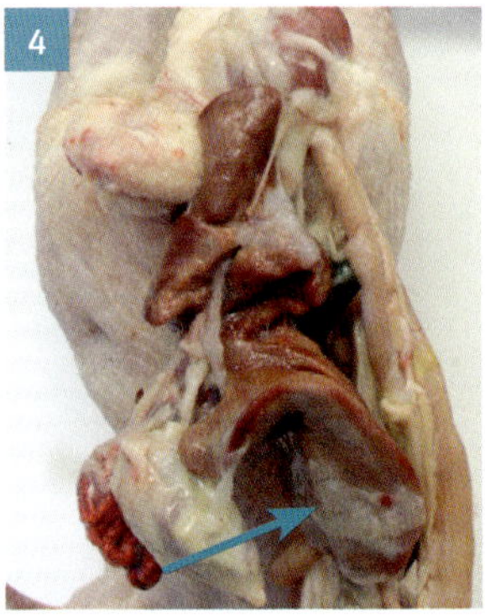

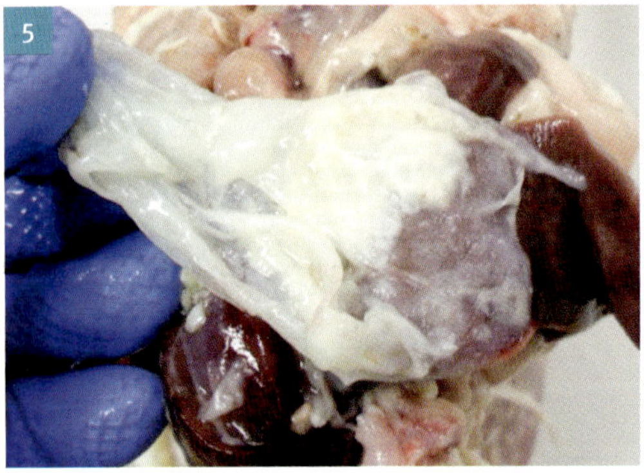

FIGURE 3. Perihepatitis. Note fibrinous tissue formation.

FIGURE 4. Classic example of perihepatitis. Note fibrous white attachments to the outside surface of the liver. Also note associated severe pericarditis. Total condemnation of the carcass and offal.

FIGURE 5. Severe perihepatitis. Note the fibrinous layer of inflammatory tissue that can be detached from the liver's surface.

Origin

Peritonitis and perihepatitis are directly related to the presence of factors which may adversely affect broiler's immune capability (Fig. 6). Such factors may include a viral infection challenge as in Marek's disease or infectious bursal disease, mycotoxines, intestinal parasites as in *Eimeria* spp., changes in feed composition and environmental conditions (dry and dusty environment, high level of ammonia or inadequate ventilation and temperature).

FIGURE 6. **Predisposing factors for the development of peritonitis and perihepatitis.**

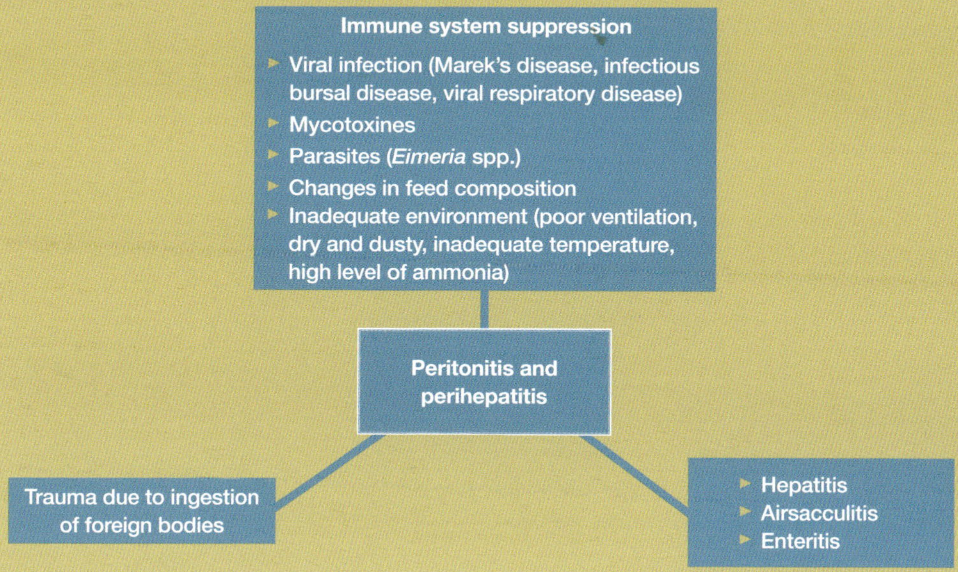

Peritonitis may be secondary to a previous condition such as hepatitis or enteritis, and also secondary to a trauma caused by the ingestion of foreign bodies. Traumatic peritonitis is uncommon in controlled intensive production systems. There is a specific form of peritonitis that affects laying hens commonly known as egg peritonitis which results from yolk material being released into the abdomen due to damaged oviducts. Egg yolk in the abdomen provides a rich medium for bacteria to thrive and cause peritonitis.

Both peritonitis and perihepatitis are normally associated with *E. coli* infection, although other bacteria such as *Pasteurella* may also be involved.

Responsibilities

All affected carcasses and associated offal are unfit for human consumption and they are consequently rejected (Figs. 7-10). The presence of peritonitis and perihepatitis makes it very difficult to judge the extent of the infection and cannot be trimmed safely. Therefore, the most sensible approach is to discard the whole carcass.

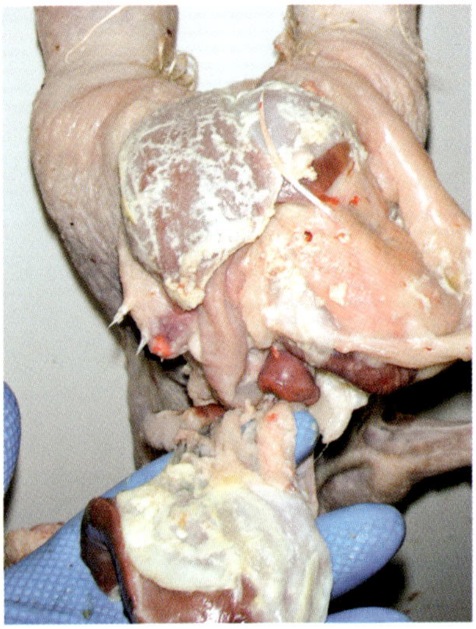

FIGURE 7. Perihepatits and peritonitis showing mucopurulent exudates. Note the fibrin on the surface of the liver. Total condemnation of the carcass and associated offal is required.

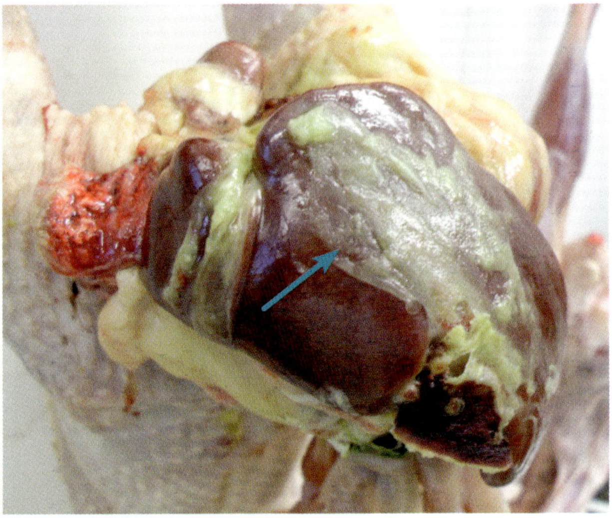

FIGURE 8. Perihepatitis to show a fibrous and dry layer of inflammatory tissue affecting the capsule of the liver. Total rejection of the carcass and associated offal.

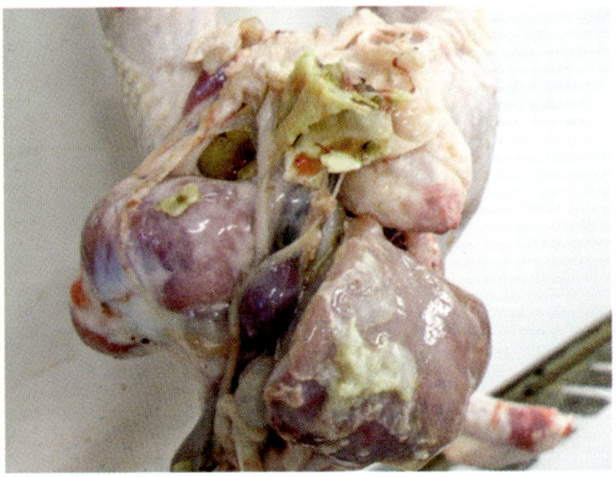

FIGURE 9. Mucopurulent perihepatitis. Total rejection of the carcass and associated offal.

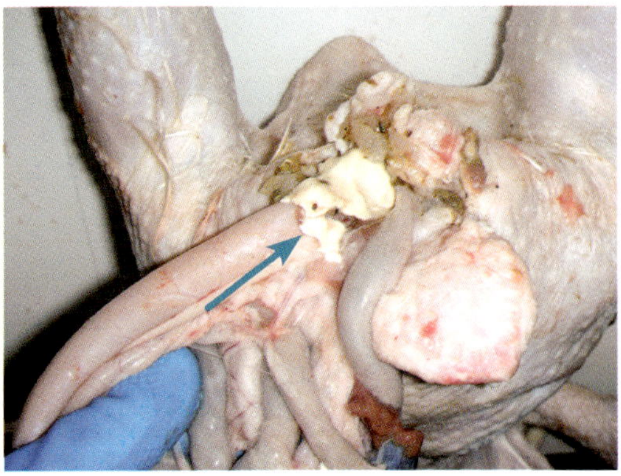

FIGURE 10. Caseous peritonitis to render carcass and offal unfit for human consumption.

Particular attention needs to be paid in high speed lines since peritonitis could easily be confused with airsacculitis. Minor peritonitis can be difficult to detect, however, perihepatitis is easy to spot while carrying out post-mortem inspection thanks to the size of the affected liver (Fig. 11). Perihepatitis is not to be confused with oedema of the liver capsule that occurs with ascitic and fevered carcasses (Fig. 12).

Reporting of this condition is extremely useful for veterinarians in the field to evaluate the health status of a given flock. It helps to determine the potential existence of an immunosuppression process due to viral challenges such as Newcastle disease or infectious bursal disease and gives an indication of the effectiveness of the vaccination programmes. It can also help the veterinary team to focus on a potential hygiene issue at the farm or in the hatchery of origin.

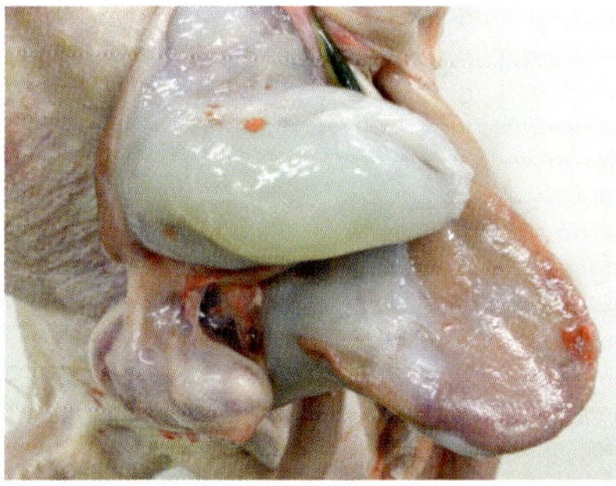

FIGURE 11. Perihepatitis associated with pericarditis.

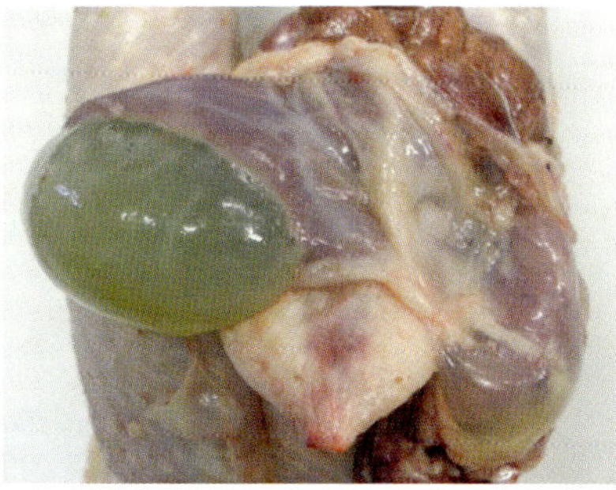

FIGURE 12. Perihepatitis and excessive accumulation of fluid within the liver capsule.

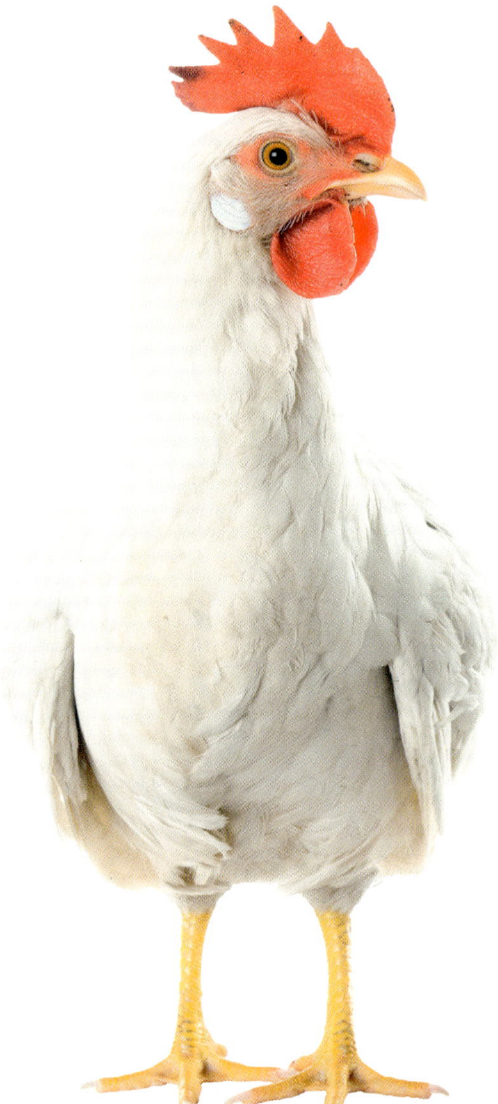

yevgeniy11/shutterstock.com

12

Ascites

Definition

Ascites is not a disease but a condition in which an abnormal quantity of fluid accumulates in the abdominal cavity (Fig. 1). Such accumulation will most frequently affect the hepatic (Fig. 2) and intestinal spaces.

Ascites is easy to identify by the inspector while carrying out post-mortem inspection due to the obvious changes in broiler's anatomy. The abdomen appears enlarged and full of fluid (Fig. 3 and 4) during whole bird inspection which can be corroborated at a later stage once evisceration has taken place.

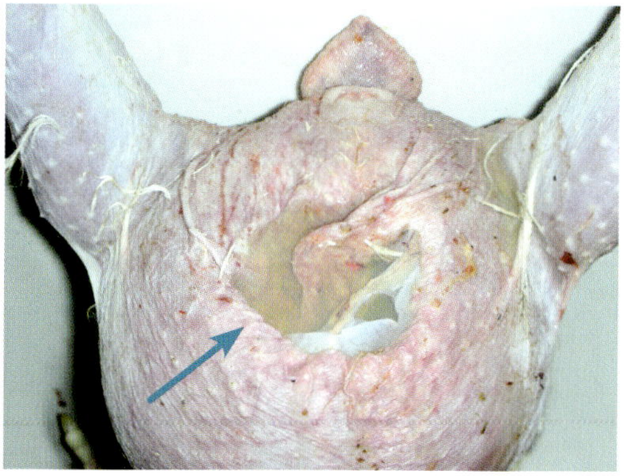

FIGURE 1. Opened carcass to show ascitic fluid in the abdomen.

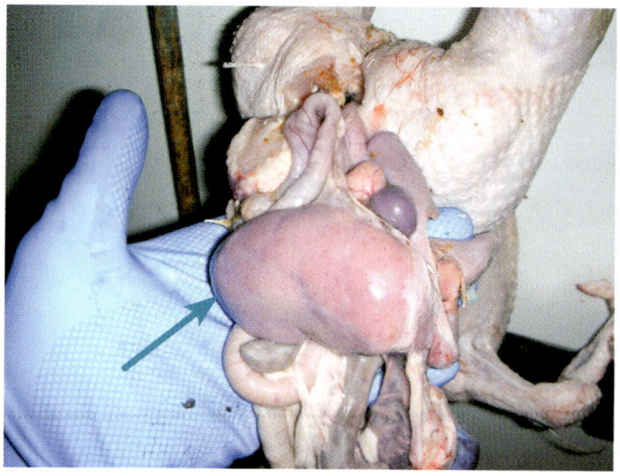

FIGURE 2. The liver is generally found pale with round edges.

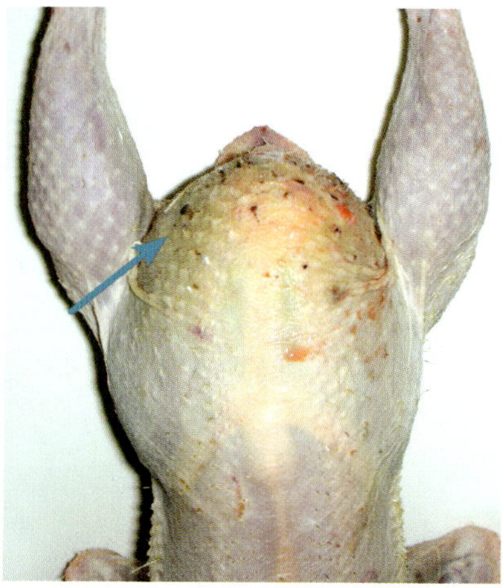

FIGURE 3. Abdomen appears enlarged due to accumulation of fluid. Note scratches affecting the abdominal area. The carcass and associated viscera were condemned as unfit for human consumption.

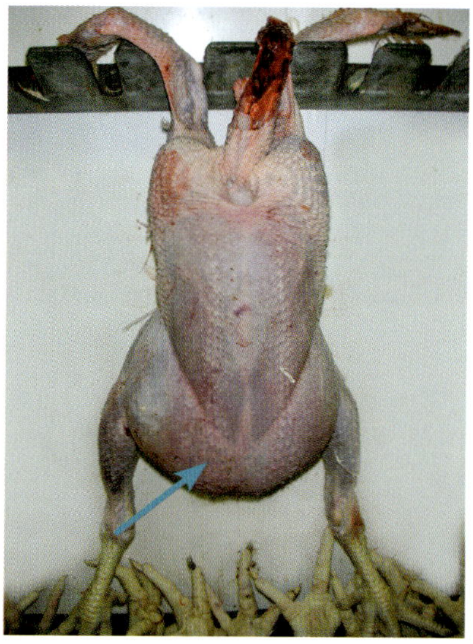

FIGURE 4. Distended abdomen due to accumulation of fluid in abdomen.

Clinically affected broilers are cyanotic and the abdominal skin may be bruised with congested peripheral vessels. Affected broilers may be of a smaller size, however, rapid growth rate is a known predisposing factor and sometimes the largest broilers are affected with occurrence in males more frequent than in females.

Ascites can be a common cause for rejection within a particular batch generally implying whole bird condemnation. Affected carcasses are normally removed while carrying out whole bird inspection.

Origin

Broilers are conditioned to a fast growth rate and they are genetically selected to achieve an amazing conversion of feed into muscle. Most of the conditions identified during post-mortem inspection are the result of a fast growth rate together with poor management at the farm.

> Ascites in broilers is mostly the result of an excessive demand for oxygen to compensate fast growth rate. Rarely due to infectious myocarditis, valvular endocarditis, degenerative disease of the myocardium or congenital heart diseases. Obstructive cholangiohepatitis caused by *Cl. perfringens* is one of the most common causes of liver damage which may also result in ascites.

An **excessive growth rate** will demand more oxygen which will increase heart rate to an extent of causing excessive pressure in pulmonary arteries. This could lead to right ventricular hypertrophy, vascular insufficiency and right ventricular failure. As a result, the liver will become congested and oedematous and fluid will leak into the abdominal body cavity to produce ascites (Figs. 5 and 6). In addition, increased demand of oxygen will prompt red blood cell production, blood thickening and circulatory flow difficultness.

There are several factors that can predispose to ascites and the most important one is air quality or adequate ventilation. Oxygen exchange is jeopardized in sheds with inadequate ventilation. Presence of dust and ammonia may irritate the lungs making oxygen use more difficult. Maintaining optimal temperature in the sheds is also critical to avoid the birds using energy and oxygen to maintain their own body temperature. All these factors may predispose a flock to ascites.

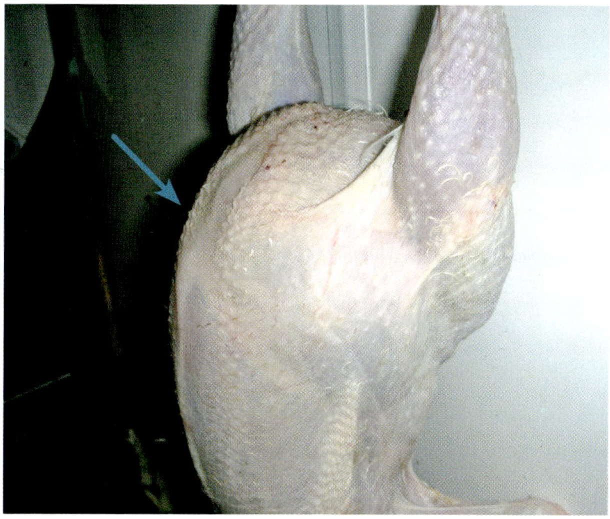

FIGURE 5. Unopened carcass showing accumulation of fluid in the abdomen.

FIGURE 6. Factors which contribute to the onset of the ascites syndrome.

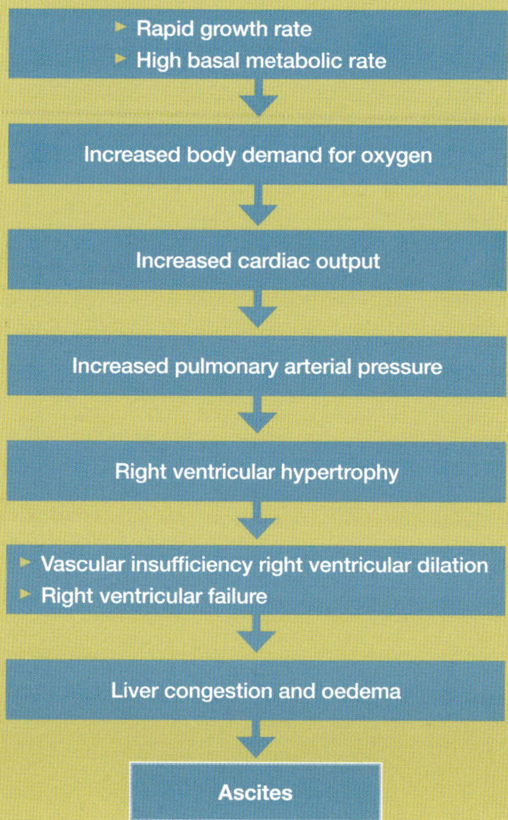

Responsibilities

Ascites in broilers is in most cases the result of a rapid growth in intensive production systems and therefore a high prevalence of ascites in a flock may have a negative impact on animal welfare. Animals with ascites are limited in movement which makes access to food more difficult. In addition, they are more prone to injury as they keep their abdomen in contact with the soil for long periods of time. Ascites in broilers is a common reason for a total rejection of the carcass and economic losses can become significant if the prevalence is high. Mild symptoms of ascites, as long as the general state of the carcass is acceptable and with no added lesions, may be considered as fit for human consumption with partial rejection of the viscera. However, author's experience is that in most cases the total rejection of the carcass is the best option.

> Affected carcasses are easily detected by the inspector prior to the point of evisceration as they usually present a swollen abdomen and in many cases signs of septicaemia. Such carcasses should, when possible, be removed prior to the evisceration process so as to avoid contamination of the machinery.

A high prevalence of ascites affecting a single batch of birds may be indicative of an animal welfare problem and therefore should be reported to the competent authority. The competent authority will then consider the history of the farm, the percentage of affected carcasses and other injuries that may indicate poor management at the farm or breaches of the relevant animal welfare regulations.

13

Septicaemia and toxaemia

Definition

Septicaemia and **toxaemia** are generalised affections caused by the presence in the bloodstream of pathogenic microorganisms or their toxins. Affected carcasses will present a darker colour through the skin with signs of dehydration and often accompanied by generalised lesions affecting internal organs of the digestive and respiratory systems (Fig. 1).

Septicaemic carcasses may show the following signs:

- A **darker meat colour** clearly seen at post-mortem inspection point (Fig. 2).
- Petechial haemorrhages on the heart, liver, kidneys, muscles and serous membranes.
- Swollen and hyperaemic liver and spleen.
- Swollen and congested kidneys.
- Hyperaemic skin.
- Muscle wasting.

Depending upon the cause and duration of septicaemia, carcasses might be hyperaemic, cyanotic, anaemic, dehydrated, oedematous, or exhibit a combination of these signs. It is important to remember that no single carcass will show all of these signs at the same time.

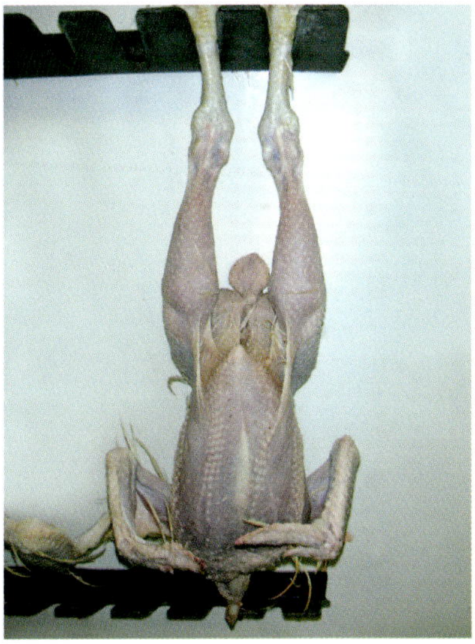

FIGURE 1. Septicaemia showing a reddish colour of the whole carcass with signs of dehydration.

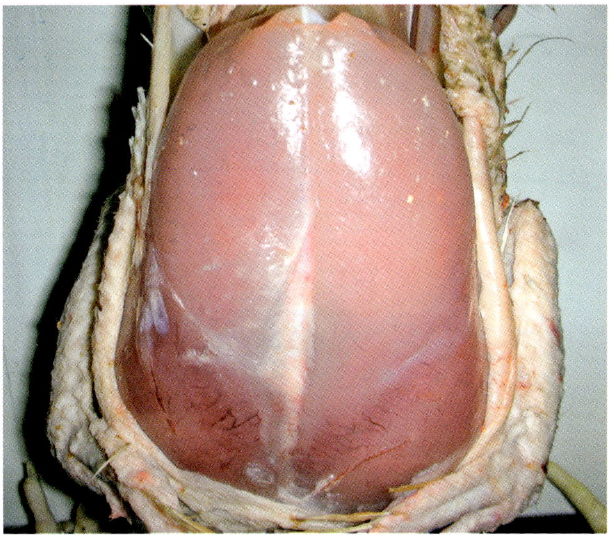

FIGURE 2. Septicaemic carcass. Note a general darker colour of the breast muscles. The carcass and associated offal are unfit for human consumption.

Origin

Septicaemia is a disease state caused by pathogenic microorganisms in the bloodstream that are able to produce systemic changes within the bird. Such changes will affect the body as a whole rather than a localised portion of it. Septicaemia and toxaemia will cause a disruption of the normal functions of the bird's organs producing a deterioration of the cells of the body. This deterioration will result in death or recovery depending on the virulence of the process and in a huge immune response which will manifest by a group of clinical signs as listed earlier in this chapter.

Toxaemia is caused by the absorption of toxins produced by pathogenic microorganisms in the body. Clinical signs are similar to septicaemia and, in fact, both conditions can coexist simultaneously.

As in most other pathological conditions, adverse environmental conditions at the farm may increase the prevalence of septicaemia and toxaemia within a flock. Viral or bacterial challenges as well as ineffective vaccines will manifest in a higher frequency of abnormal colour carcasses at post-mortem inspection. The health status of the flock is consequently directly related to the frequency of septicaemic carcasses at slaughter.

Responsibilities

The meat inspector will not be able to differentiate between septicaemia and toxaemia at post-mortem inspection. In any case, **all affected carcasses and offal are condemned** and they are unfit for human consumption.

> Special attention needs to be paid to carcasses showing a bright and reddish colour which could be mistaken for septicaemia. The skin and feather follicles are very sensitive to temperature changes, particularly in adverse weather, which can produce hyperaemia of the skin. Older broiler birds tend to be more susceptible to hyperaemia of the skin than younger birds. Such carcasses are perfectly fit for human consumption and should not be mistaken for septicaemic or poorly bled carcasses. Note that septicaemic carcasses would normally appear dehydrated, soft to the touch and generally but not always showing poor general condition.

Identifying septicaemia and toxaemia requires experience and concentration, although the majority of cases are easy to identify at whole bird inspection point (Figs. 3-6). Checking the elasticity of the skin while looking for signs of dehydration may help to properly diagnose the condition.

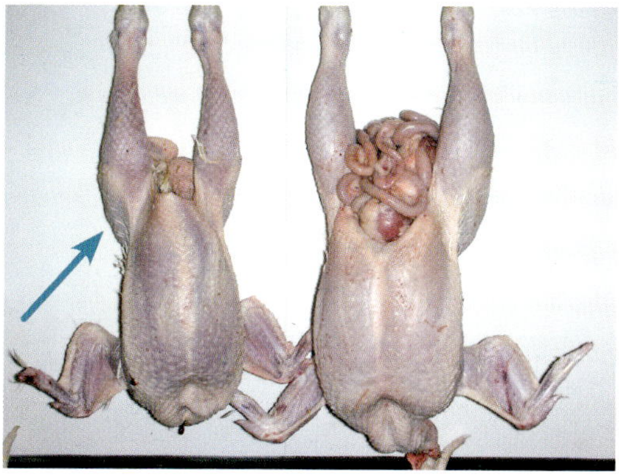

FIGURE 3. Septicaemic carcass (arrowed) compared to a fit carcass.

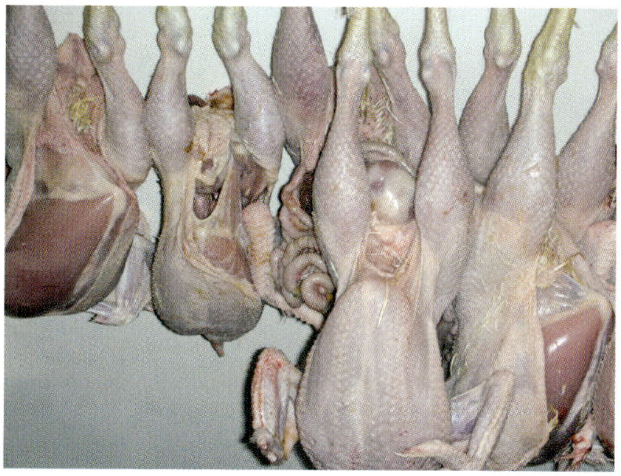

FIGURE 4. Batch of birds severely affected by septicaemia or toxaemia.

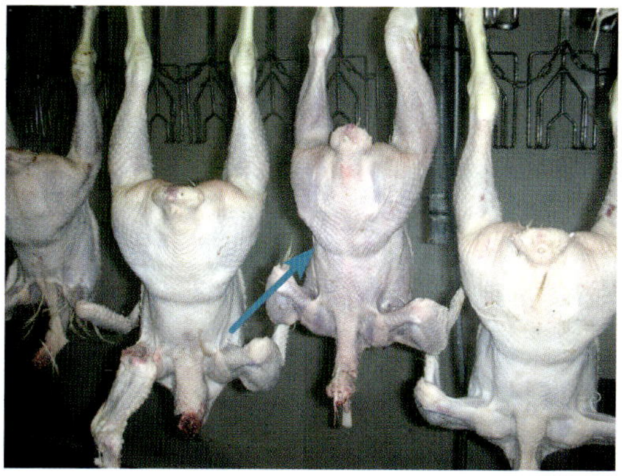

FIGURE 5. Septicaemic carcass identified at whole bird inspection point (arrow). Note the difference in colour compared to other carcasses.

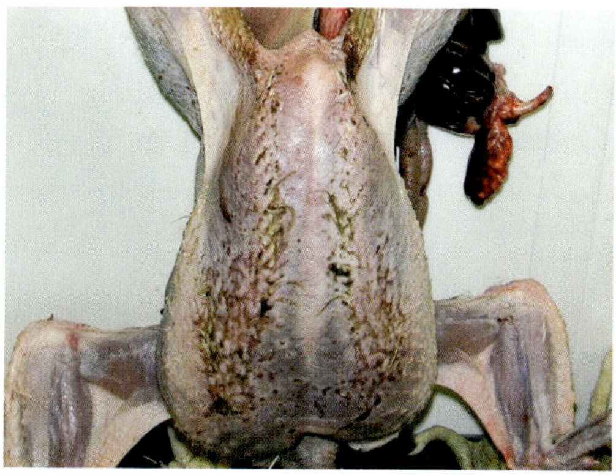

FIGURE 6. Septicaemia, more frequently seen when slaughtering batches of birds, showing poor general condition and dermatitis.

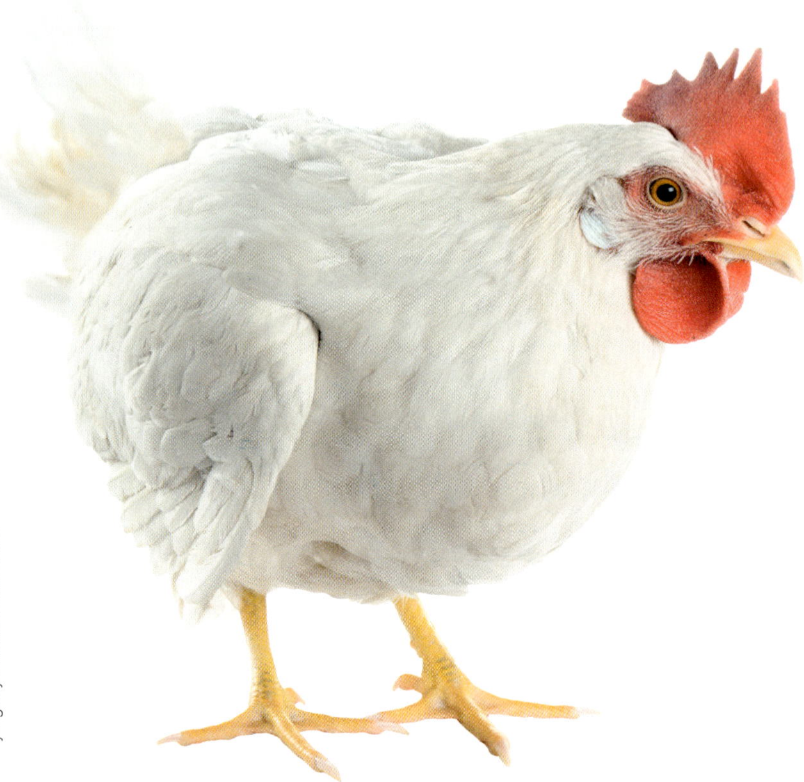

yevgeniy11/shutterstock.com

14

Other pathologies

Pendulous crop

Pendulous crop is a condition in which the crop appears excessively enlarged due to accumulation of fluid, feed and litter (Fig. 1).

The aetiology is not known although there are studies suggesting a hereditary predisposition and an exacerbation of the condition due to erratic or excessive feed or water consumption. Food impaction blocking the alimentary tract may eventually result in accumulation of feed and fluid in the crop, and it is not uncommon to see food impaction of the proventriculus and ventriculus associated with pendulous crop (Fig. 2). Vagus nerve damage has also been postulated as a cause. Affected birds may have their feeding capabilities impaired and become thin or emaciated.

Pendulous crop is relatively rare at post-mortem inspection. Affected carcasses are ideally removed from the line before entering the evisceration machinery to avoid any potential cross contamination or machine damage. Such carcasses are often trimmed manually under the supervision of a veterinarian or a qualified inspector and then passed as fit for human consumption if there are no other associated lesions. Carcasses showing poor general condition, septicaemia, abnormal odour or emaciation should be condemned.

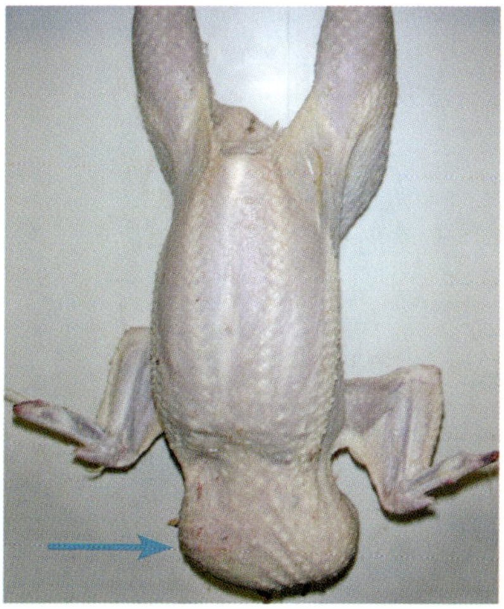

FIGURE 1. Pendulous crop affecting a broiler carcass. Such carcasses are removed when possible prior to entering the evisceration machinery so as to avoid any risk of cross contamination and machine damage. Affected carcasses are passed as fit for human consumption when there are no other associated conditions observed.

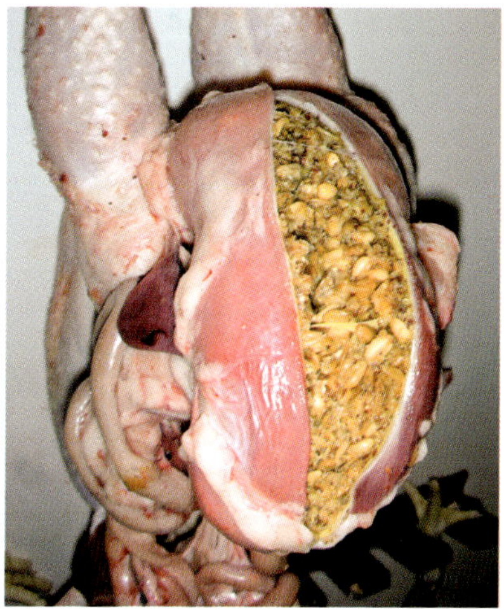

FIGURE 2. Food impaction of the proventriculus and ventriculus in a carcass also affected by pendulous crop.

Badly bled

After stunning or stun-killing, the bleeding of birds is the final stage of the slaughter process. Bleeding, also referred to as neck-cutting, may be undertaken either manually with a sharp knife or by use of an automated rotating neck cutter. The cut must sever at least one of the carotid arteries or the vessels from which they arise. More rapid bleeding-out is achieved if both carotid arteries are cut.

It is a legal requirement that bleeding must be undertaken without delay after any bird is stunned (or stun-killed). The time between stunning and bleeding must be as short as possible. Once neck cutting has occurred, birds must be left for a period of time (90 seconds according to European legislation) in order to ensure that it is dead before further processing can take place.

Badly bled carcasses are identified at the post-mortem inspection point and characterised by general cherry red skin affecting particularly the neck region and congestion of blood vessels and organs caused as a result of the insufficient bleeding of the carcass (Figs. 1-3).

Poor bleeding may be due to bad sticking practices or poor automatic neck cutter performance. Badly bled carcasses need to be monitored since they can result in a breach of the Animal Welfare Regulations. Judgement means that carcasses and offal are unfit for human consumption.

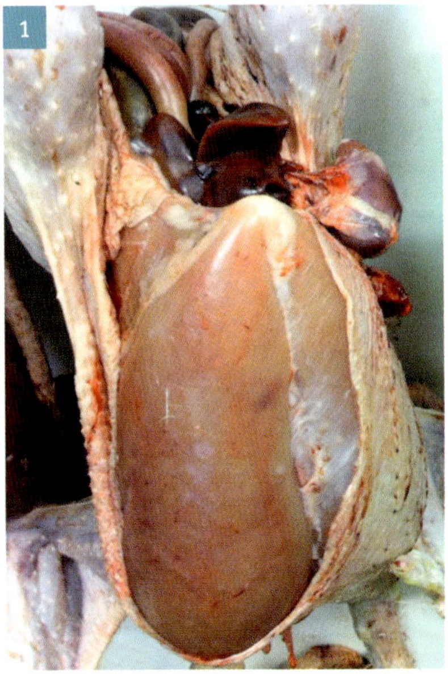

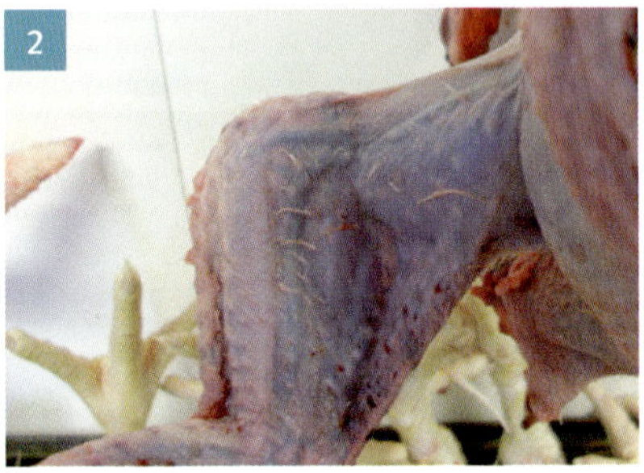

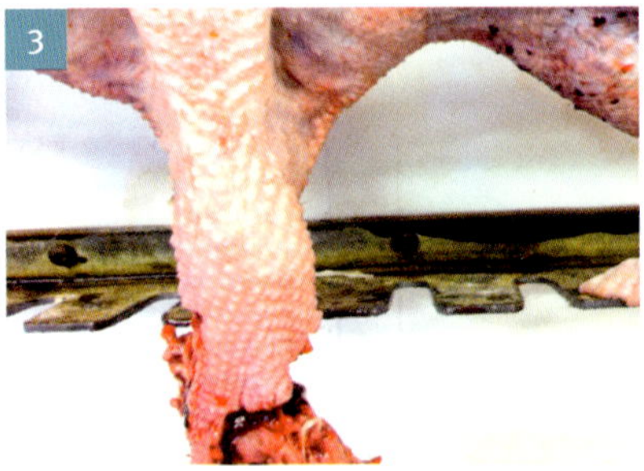

FIGURE 1. Poorly bled carcass. Note congested breast muscles and wings. Carcass and associated offal are unfit for human consumption. Animal welfare could be compromised at this point when stun to stun is performed as stunning method since the bird could recover consciousness prior to entering the scalding tanks.

FIGURE 2. Congested wings due to poor bleeding.

FIGURE 3. Note redness of the neck indicating poor bleeding.

Anasarca

Anasarca is characterised by an accumulation of fluid in the subcutaneous area under the skin that can be described as a jelly-like consistency (Fig. 1). This condition is rare but renders the carcass unfit for human consumption. It is often seen in conjunction with ascitis and its origin is not certain. Several studies relate it to vascular damage as a result of the presence of toxins or due to inadequate diets and particularly due to an insufficiency in vitamin E.

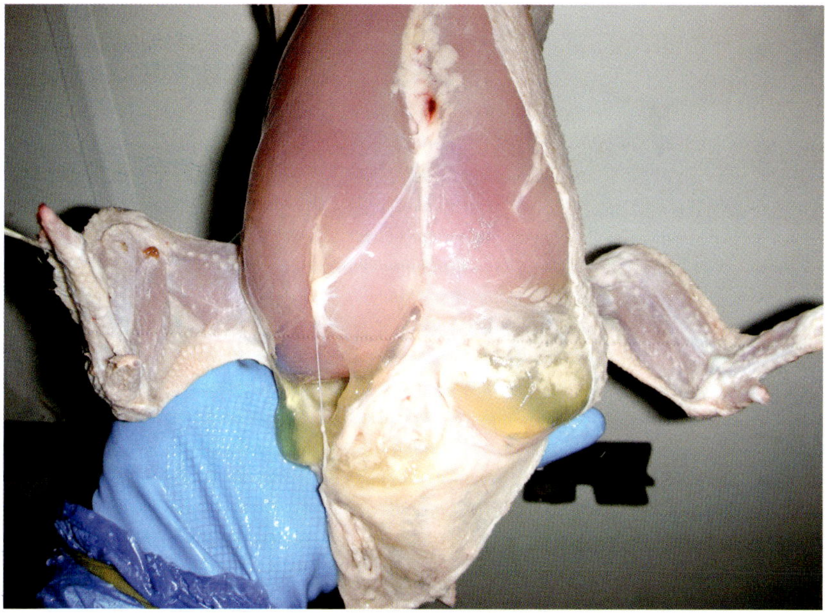

FIGURE 1. Anasarca will normally affect the breast, wings and back.

Nutritional muscular dystrophy or white muscle disease

This disease is normally associated with a mineral deficiency and it is characterised by a white striped pattern in the muscle, more evident in the breast (Fig. 1). According to several studies, it occurs in the presence of combined deficiencies of selenium and vitamin E. A deficiency of sulphur amino acids also contributes to the development of the disease. This myopathy affects more commonly the superficial pectoral muscles, the abductor wing muscles and occasionally the skeletal muscles of the torso. Affected carcasses are unfit for human consumption.

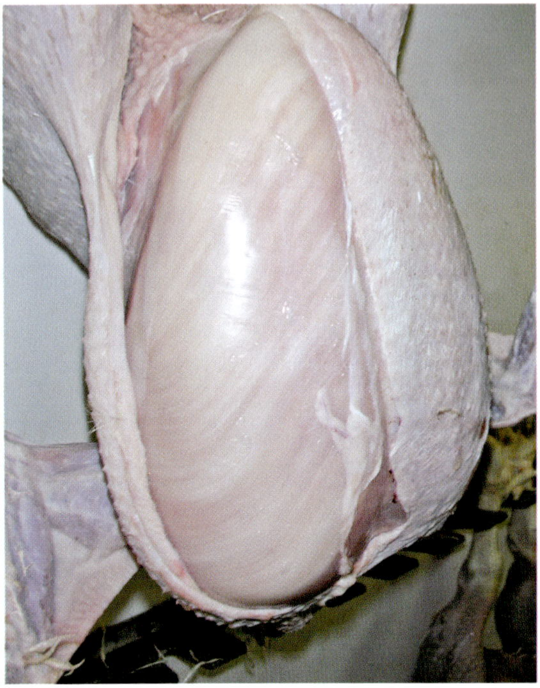

FIGURE 1. Suspected white muscle disease in a broiler carcass.

Ruptured gastrocnemius tendon or green leg

Ruptured gastrocnemius tendons are common within broiler intensive production systems, particularly in older broilers and breeders. This condition is commonly known as green leg and may be unilateral or bilateral (Fig. 1). The gastrocnemius tendon is located at the rear of the hock and can snap due to a number of reasons resulting in bruising of the leg that will turn green as the bruising ages. As the tendon separates prior to rupture, the tendon and tendon sheath are frequently thickened by fibroplasia and other repair processes.

This condition may be the result of the bird's bodyweight together with poor tendon development. It is thought that rapid growth may result in poor blood supply and avascular degeneration resulting in poor tendon strength. A viral or bacterial tenosynovitis may also result in ruptured gastrocnemius tendons.

Affected carcasses are fit for human consumption providing that trimming of the affected parts is carried out hygienically. The Food Business Operator should have a trimming policy in place to deal with green leg disease and in particular those premises processing older broilers or breeders.

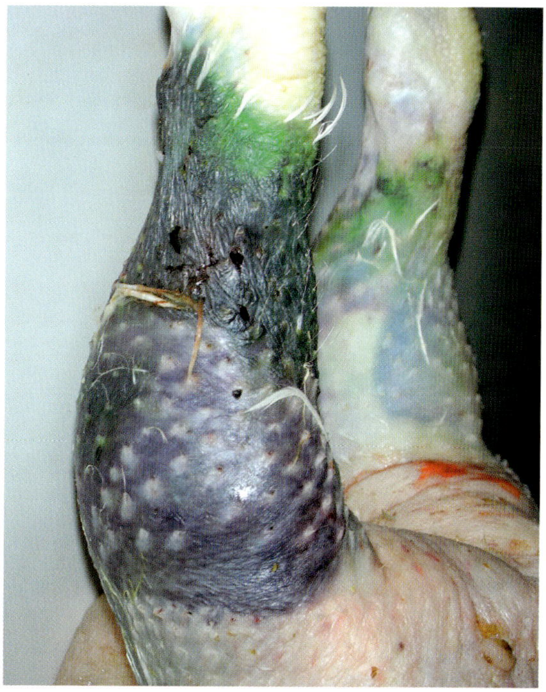

FIGURE 1. Bilateral ruptured gastrocnemius tendon also known as green leg disease. Rest of the carcass can be salvaged.

Oregon disease

Oregon disease is defined as a non-infectious ischaemic necrosis of the deep pectoral muscle. This condition is also known as green muscle disease or deep pectoral myopathy. It does not usually cause any mortality or obvious clinical signs and so it is usually identified after slaughter. Prevalence is higher in turkeys than in broiler birds.

Oregon disease is caused by a reduction of the blood supply to the deep pectoral muscles, and particularly to the supracoracoideus muscle. Genetics may play a role in that it has been suggested that blood supply to the affected muscles is reduced in some heavy meat type birds. The condition can be reproduced by causing intense exercise of this muscle. Because it is enclosed in a relatively unyielding membrane, any swelling of the muscle tends to cut off the blood supply. Without adequate blood supply, the tissue of the muscle begins to die, or suffer necrosis.

Oregon disease is not detected at post-mortem inspection point since lesions only affect the deep pectoral muscle and so it is detected during further processing of the carcass in cutting plants.

Breast blister

Commonly found when processing batches of birds that have been affected by a wet or caked litter. Breast blister is defined as a swelling over the keel bone accompanied by bruising and discolouration of the skin (Fig. 1). The inflammation of the skin will give way to scar tissue in more chronic cases. Infection by *Staphylococcus* is common but lesions are localised and not fatal. Affected carcasses are normally passed as fit for human consumption and trimmed accordingly. Carcasses showing generally poor condition and extensive skin damaged are condemned as unfit for human consumption.

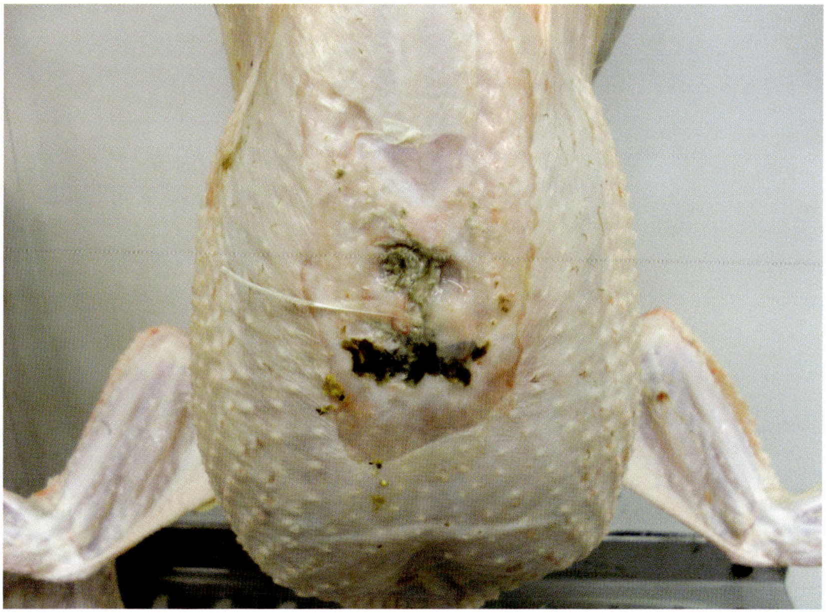

FIGURE 1. Breast blister.

Enteritis

Enteritis refers to the inflammation of the small intestine.

Two well-known forms of enteritis are ulcerative enteritis, caused by *Cl. colinum*, and necrotic enteritis, caused by *Cl. perfringens*. *Clostridia* are highly resistant to environmental factors and are found in soil, dirt, manure and in small quantities in the intestine of healthy chickens. The bacterium only causes disease when it proliferates in large numbers, producing extracellular toxins that attack the intestines of birds, causing injury. Such injuries vary depending on the virulence of the infection and they can be characterised by thickening of the intestinal wall and dark brown contents with necrotic material (Fig. 1). The intestines of infected birds can also be friable and distended with gas and gross lesions caused by the toxins (Fig. 2).

Certain forms of enteritis may result from excess heat, cold, overcrowded houses, deficient intake of food materials, coccidiosis or toxic substances.

Enteritis is judged upon general condition of the carcass. Partial rejection of the offal is possible when there are no other associated conditions or signs of systemic disorder.

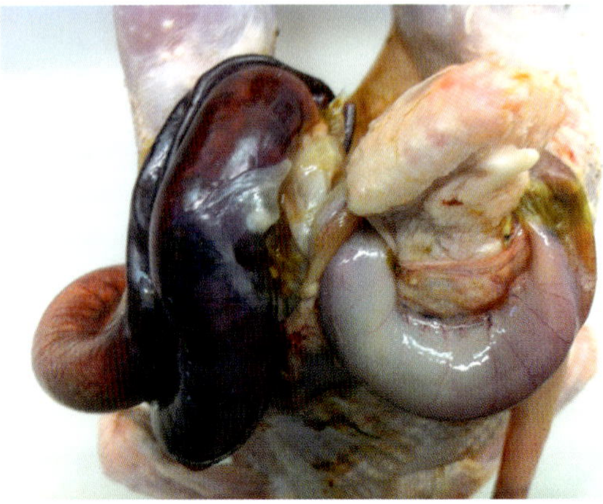

FIGURE 1. Enteritis characterised by dark brown contents with possible necrotic material and congested intestinal walls.

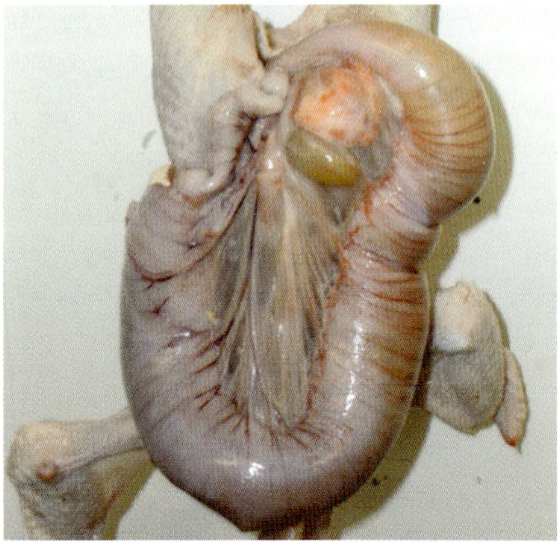

FIGURE 2. Distended intestines with watery or foamy contents.

Fatty liver syndrome

Fatty liver syndrome is described as excessive fat in the liver occasionally associated with various degrees of haemorrhage. The condition is almost universally confined to caged birds fed high energy diets, and is most often seen in summer months. The liver is usually enlarged, yellow and very friable with an abdominal cavity containing large amounts of fat. Fatty liver syndrome without excessive body fat is thought to be associated with mycotoxins (e.g., aflatoxins) in feed (Fig. 1).

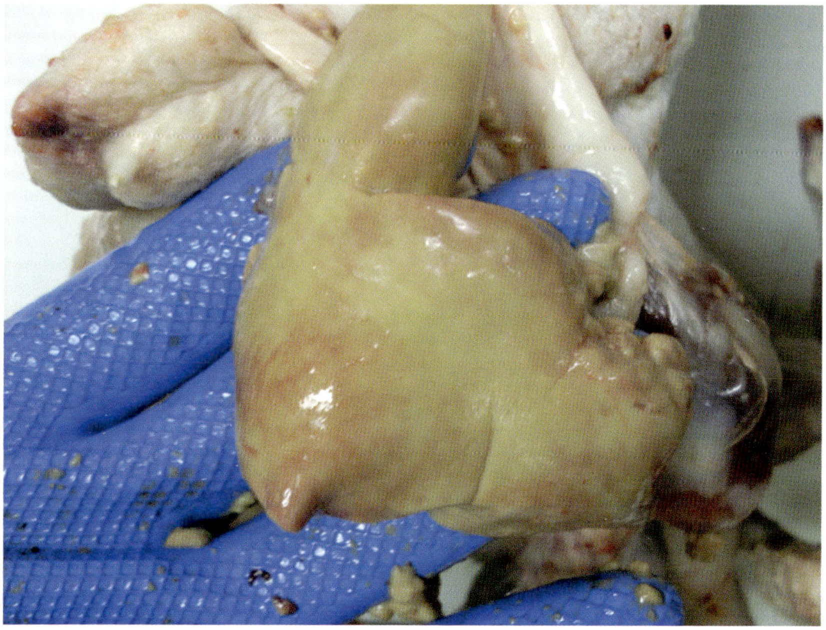

FIGURE 1. Suspected fatty liver syndrome in a broiler possibly caused by mycotoxins. Partial rejection of the offal only.

Tumours

It is thought that the most common tumours found at post-mortem inspection in broilers are caused by **Marek's disease**. However, diagnosis of lymphoid tumours in poultry is complicated due to multiple aetiological agents capable of causing very similar tumours. It is not uncommon that more than one avian tumour virus can be present in a chicken. Marek's disease is a highly contagious viral neoplastic disease in chickens caused by an *alphaherpesvirus*, known as Marek's disease virus or *Gallid herpesvirus 2* (GaHV-2). This disease may result in lymphomatous tumours that could affect multiple areas of the carcass such the skin, the skeletal muscles and visceral organs such the ovary, spleen (Fig. 1), liver, kidneys, lungs, heart, proventriculus and adrenals.

Avian sarcoma leukosis virus can also cause a wide range of tumours being lymphomas the most common type. The disease is also characterised by an enlarged liver due to infiltration of cancerous lymphoid cells. In addition, other abdominal organs and the bursa of Fabricius are often infected. This disease cannot be differentiated from other viral diseases at post-mortem inspection point.

Haemangiomas are benign tumours caused by congenital overgrowth of the blood vessels that may occur in the skin or internal organs. Bleeding is not uncommon and may be significant following injury to the haemangioma.

Other tumours include keratoacanthomas, adenocarcinomas and fibromas:

- **Keratoacanthomas,** also known as **squamous cell carcinomas,** are skin tumours that arise from the feather follicle of the skin and are relatively common at post-mortem inspection. These tumours are multicentric in nature, which means that they can arise in different areas on the bird but are still considered to be benign (Figs. 2 and 3).
- **Adenocarcinomas** are tumours derived from glandular tissue or in which the tumour cells form recognizable glandular structures. They normally affect abdominal organs and are common in older birds.
- **Fibromas** may develop in any connective tissue. They are more common also in older birds.

Numerous other types of tumours occur in domestic poultry but at a low frequency.

Carcasses are generally condemned for tumours if there is gross evidence of metastasis (more than one tumour of the same kind indicating spread), or if one large tumour causes a systemic disruption.

> Condemned young chickens showing generalised signs of avian keratoacanthoma with large coalescence, joining together lesions. Trimming may be possible when lesions are localised or if only a few small keratoacanthoma lesions are present.

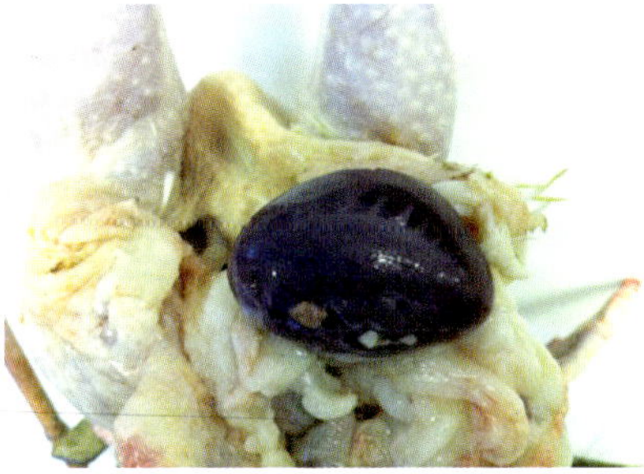

FIGURE 1. Tumour of the spleen. The carcass was also showing poor general condition resulting in total rejection.

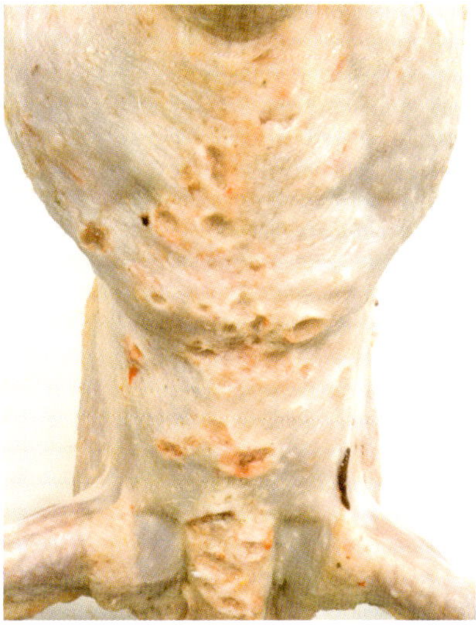

FIGURE 2. Keratoacanthoma affecting the skin of a broiler carcass. Total condemnation considering the extension of the tumour.

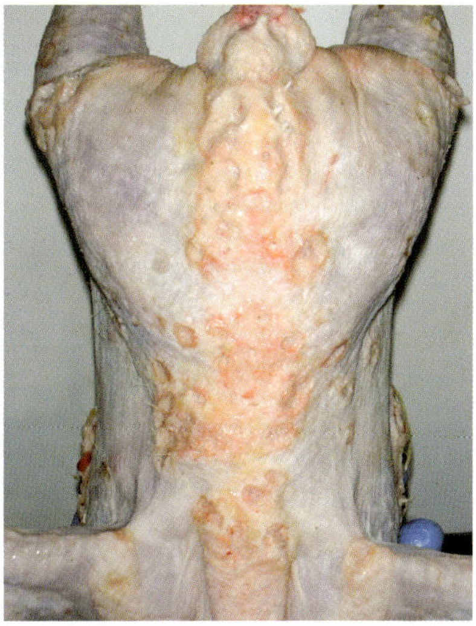

FIGURE 3. Extensive keratoacanthoma resulting in total carcass condemnation.

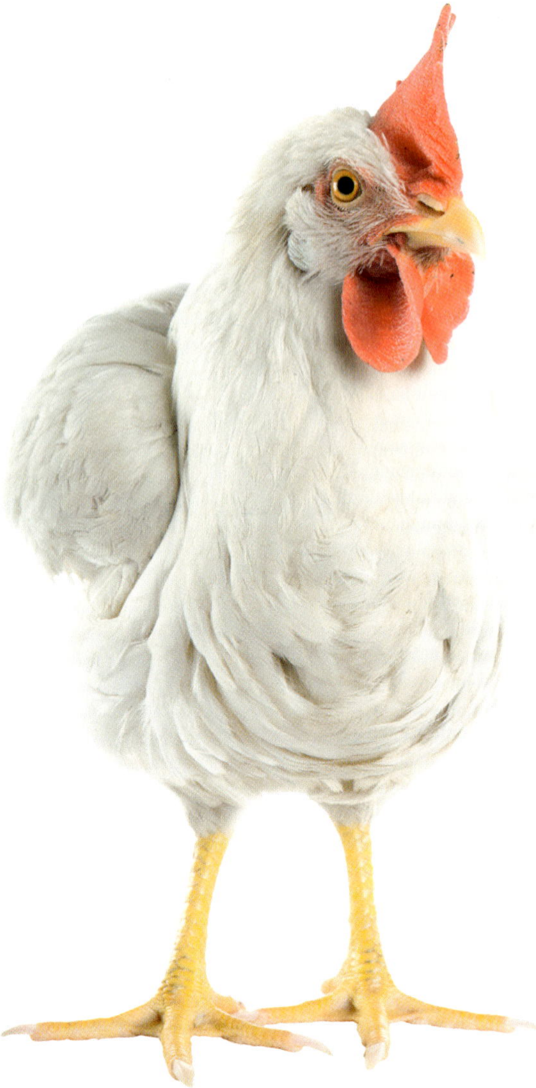

15

Others

Poultry feet and offal for human consumption

Feet harvested for human consumption must come from birds that have been passed fit for human consumption at post-mortem (Figs. 1-3). The feet themselves must be inspected. Inspection of the feet may take place at the whole bird inspection stage provided the harvesting systems ensure that the feet from birds rejected at evisceration are not collected for human consumption. Alternatively, feet can be inspected later, at the pre-packing stage, again provided that the feet from any rejected bird are not included in those processed for human consumption.

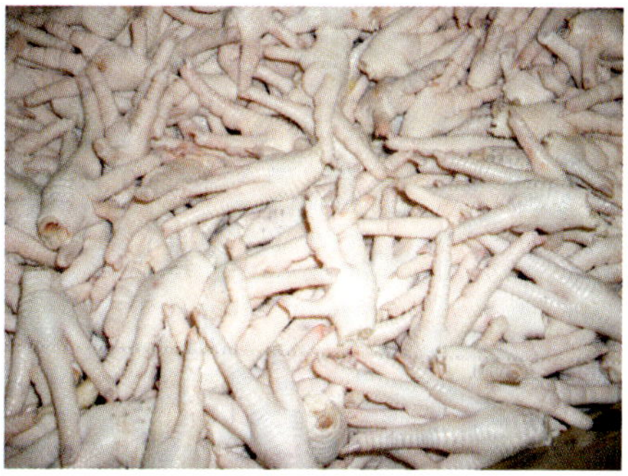

FIGURE 1. Feet harvested for human consumption.

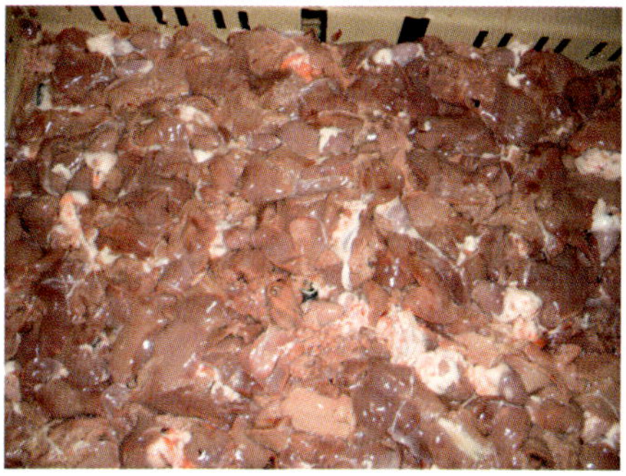

FIGURE 2. Livers being collected to be sold as fit for human consumption. Routine checks should be undertaken by the veterinarian or inspector to ensure that the harvesting of livers is carried out hygienically with no signs of visible contamination.

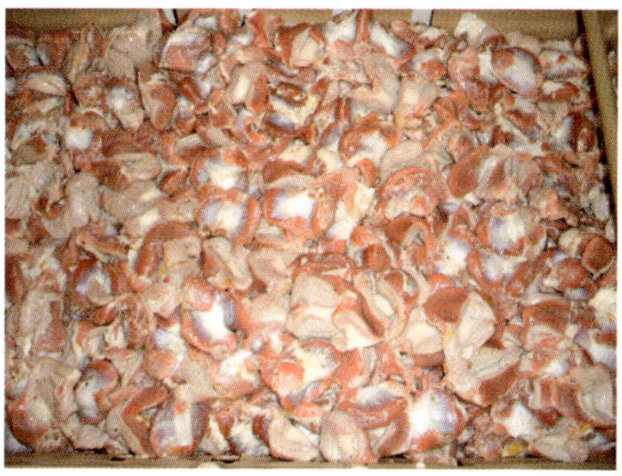

FIGURE 3. Gizzards need to be inspected to verify that all surfaces have been thoroughly cleaned to show no visible signs of digestive contents.

Other rejections due to poor processing

Overscalding

Overscalded carcasses are those that spend too much time in the scald tank to become partially or totally cooked. This usually occurs due to a breakdown of the automated line (Fig. 1), although there are other possible causes such as poor adjustment of the scald tank temperature or improper line speed. Carcasses are characterised by a cooked appearance, the skin feels slimy and the underlying meat is much whiter than usual. The skin and meat become more friable and often machine damaged as they pass the plucking machines.

Overscalded carcasses and associated offal are condemned due to the added risk of cross contamination during the scalding and plucking processes, and also due to the organoleptic changes caused to the meat. Slightly overscalded carcasses may be salvaged but this needs to be in accordance with an effective trimming policy and under the supervision of the meat inspection team. Always refer to current legislation in force with regards to trimming procedures of overscalded carcasses if any.

The Food Business Operator shall have a contingency plan to the satisfaction of the veterinarian to properly identify overscalded carcasses in the event of a breakdown of the automated line.

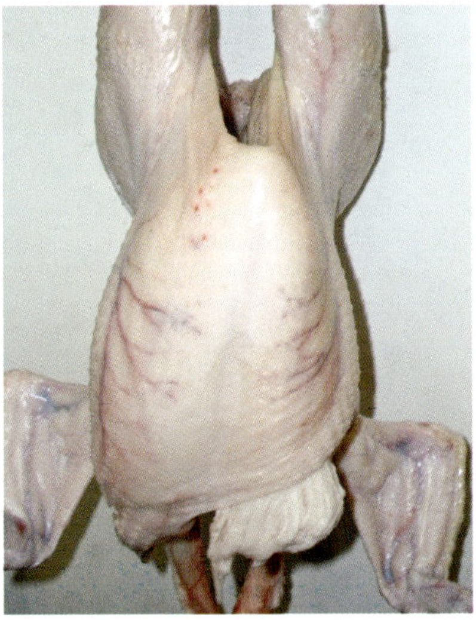

FIGURE 1. Overscalded carcass due to a breakdown of the automated line. Note cooked appearance of the meat. Total condemnation of the carcass and associated offal.

Poor plucking

Poor plucking is a factory related condition in which an excessive number of feathers are left on the carcasses due to ineffective plucking procedures (Fig. 1).

The most probable causes of poor plucking are:

- Temperature too low in scalding tanks.
- Poor maintenance of plucking machine.
- Inadequate setting of the plucking machines in relation to the bird's size.
- Inadequate line speed.

Remaining feathers are a source of contamination at later stages in the production line, particularly after the chilling process, since once carcasses have been chilled they are placed in boxes or baskets or sent to a cutting plant for further processing. Feathers are therefore a source of contamination to all contact surfaces and to other carcasses.

Affected carcasses would not necessary need to be discarded and can be detained to be reworked although this needs to be carried out without delay. The Food Business Operator shall put a system in place to monitor plucking standards and to ensure that corrective action is taken when needed.

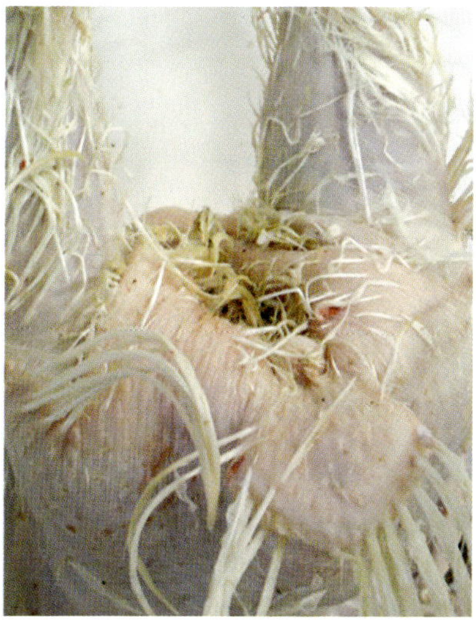

FIGURE 1. Poorly plucked carcass reveals an excessive amount of feathers left after the plucking process. Such carcasses are allowed to be removed from the line to be reworked providing that such action is taken without delay. Feathers are a source of contamination to contact surfaces and to other carcasses and therefore need to be removed prior to the chilling process. Carcasses that are not rectified promptly or those beyond rectification are condemned as unfit for human consumption.

Contamination

Definition

Contamination refers to the presence in food of harmful chemicals and microorganisms. The most common sources of contamination are faecal contamination, bilis contamination and chemical contamination (grease, disinfectants, etc.).

Origin

When automated lines are used, poor alignment of the evisceration machines may result in damage to the digestive tract and subsequent spillage of gut contents with contamination of the carcass. Adequate maintenance and adjustment of the machinery to the size of birds is important to avoid this. Pluckers that are not cleaned properly on a daily basis or well-maintained may contaminate carcasses with grease and dirt, and also cause damage to the skin leaving the meat unprotected to become contaminated (Fig. 1).

When manual evisceration is carried out, contamination can be caused by infrequent rinsing and disinfecting of knives or inadequate washing of the operative's arms and hands.

Broilers must be off-feed prior to slaughter to reduce the risk of faecal contamination during processing and evisceration. Different research results confirm that the best gastrointestinal clean-out is achieved when broilers are kept off-feed for 8-12 hours before hanging. As the digestion cycle commonly takes about 6 hours to conclude, broilers kept off-feed for less than 8 hours have an increased

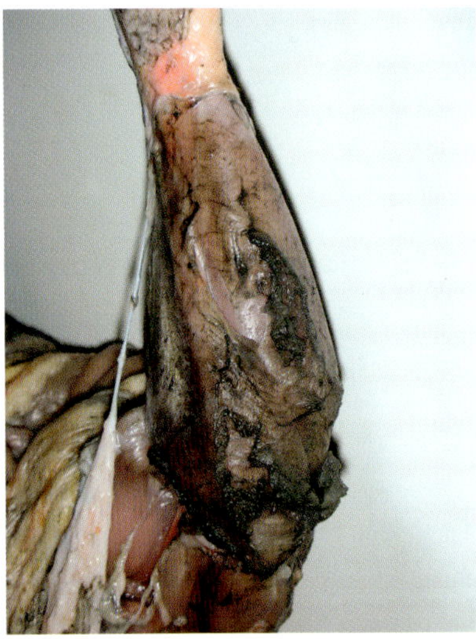

FIGURE 1. Grease contamination affecting unprotected fresh meat. Condemnation of the affected part is required.

likelihood of being contaminated by either faeces or digestive content during the manual or, particularly, the automatic evisceration (Fig. 2). Likewise, broilers off-feed for more than 12 hours are also subject to contamination, yet of different nature, during evisceration. In this case their intestines undergo a degradation of the epithelium, which results in the loosening of its mechanical strength. Weakened, the intestines can be easily torn during evisceration, allowing its content - not faeces, but the fluids resulting from the epithelial degradation - to spill onto the carcasses. Additionally, broilers deprived of feed and water for such periods of time experience significant and irreversible live weight shrinkage prior to slaughter.

Responsibilities

Carcasses that are contaminated to the extent that valid inspection cannot be made are condemned. An example would be a carcass contaminated with bile or faeces to the extent that the inspector cannot determine whether the carcass is wholesome.

Carcasses that are mishandled and fall into open sewers or evisceration troughs are also condemned under the contamination category (Fig. 3). Such carcasses should not be passed as fit for human consumption since the degree of contamination cannot be determined. These contaminated carcasses are the result of an improper adjustment of the machinery in relation to the size of the birds, or due to poor maintenance of the machinery. The responsibility includes reporting any unusual number of carcasses being condemned for contamination during processing, since this is valuable information to the Food Business Operator as part of their maintenance and quality control checks.

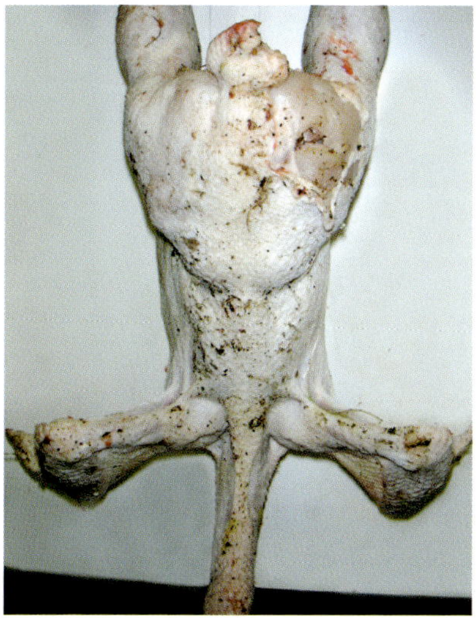

FIGURE 2. Extensive faecal contamination affecting a carcass with some skin damage to expose fresh meat. Total condemnation was required.

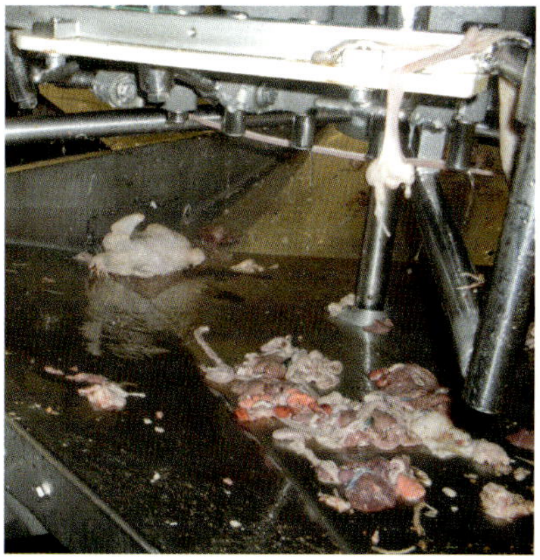

FIGURE 3. Carcasses may fall into the working machinery of the evisceration room becoming contaminated and occasionally blocking the drains of the machines.

Any part of the carcass or offal affected with bile staining should be trimmed. Where plucking machines break the skin of poultry, the underlying musculature should be considered to be contaminated and trimmed from the carcass (Fig. 4). Meat contaminated after post-mortem inspection must not be released for human consumption.

The Food Business Operator is to ensure that any sort of contamination is avoided prior to the chilling process (Fig. 5). Any contamination detected thereafter needs to be removed in accordance with a trimming policy and under the supervision of a veterinarian or a qualified inspector. Recording and reporting of such findings is paramount to determine the level of contamination that affects a particular plant and to evaluate the need of enforcement to address a potential maintenance or operational issue and to safeguard the wholesomeness of the final product.

The inspector or veterinarian will pay special attention to several factors in the event of a high level of contamination on carcasses (Fig. 6). Irregular batches of birds may increase contamination levels due the impossibility of adjusting the machinery to different sizes of birds simultaneously. The Food Business Operator shall take pertinent corrective action when processing a bad batch of birds in order to avoid any contamination entering the chillers, normally increasing manpower and reducing the speed of the line.

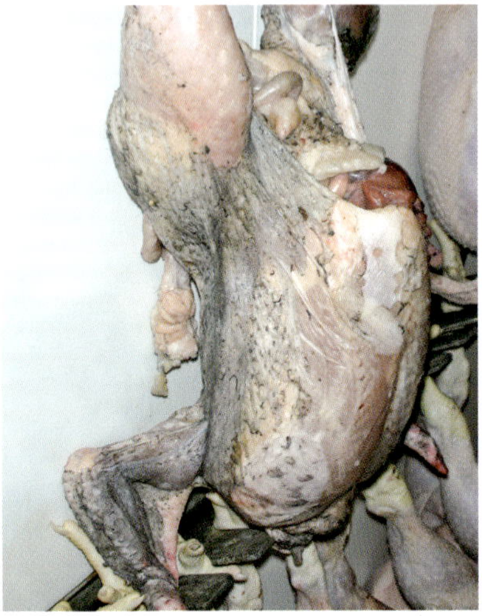

FIGURE 4. Extensive skin contamination due to improper use of the plucking machine. Commonly seen when pluckers are being left running with an empty line for several minutes. Total rejection.

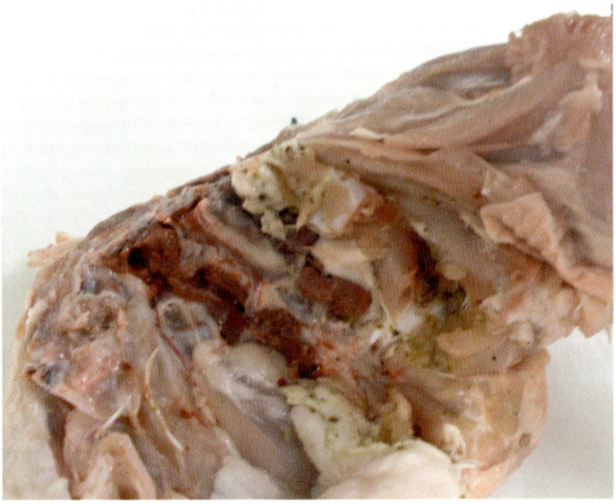

FIGURE 5. Note faecal contamination affecting the inguinal area of a carcass due to poor evisceration or machine damage during production.

Figure 6. Factors to take into account by the inspector or veterinarian in the event of a high level of contamination on carcasses.

- Improper adjustment of the evisceration machines
- Poor maintenance of the evisceration machines
- Poor cleaning of the plucking machines
- Poor operational practices when manually eviscerated
- Feed withdrawal period not met
- Slaughter of an irregular batch of birds/uneven sizes
- Inadequate preoperational and operational cleanings standards of the evisceration machines

Machine damage and bruising

Definition

This chapter includes any physical alteration to the carcass before and during processing at the abattoir.

Bruising can be defined as a type of haematoma of tissue in which capillaries and sometimes venules are damaged by trauma, allowing blood to seep into the surrounding interstitial tissues.

Generally known as machine damage carcasses are those which include any physical alteration caused by machinery during processing (Fig. 1).

Luxations occur when bones in a joint become displaced or misaligned, but fractures will be referred when there is a break in the continuity of the bone. Luxations and fractures can also be included in machine damage when the condition is caused by machinery during processing.

Damage of carcasses that may be caused during the processing must be differentiated from damage to the live bird. The most frequent injuries are bruises, broken limbs and damaged wings.

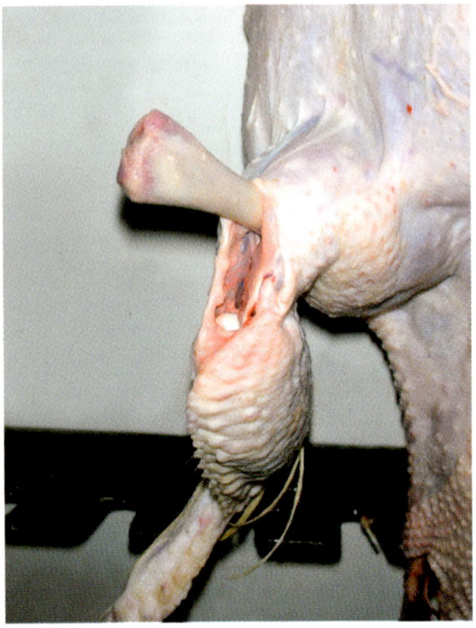

FIGURE 1. Broken wings are the most common machine damage condition found during post-mortem inspection.

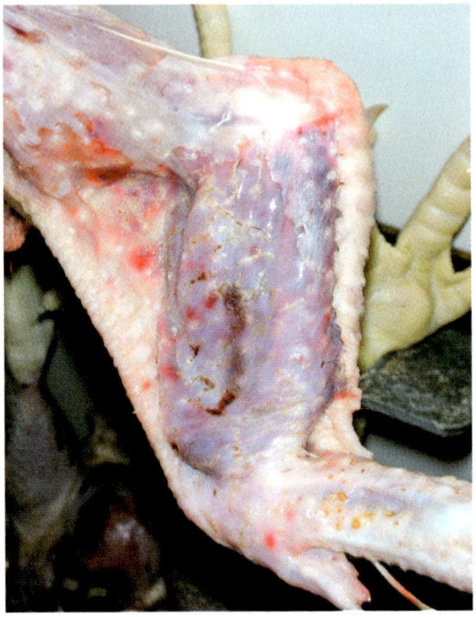

FIGURE 2. Recently bruised wing. Bright redness to indicate a fresh bruise with free blood under the skin.

Origin

Poultry bruises result from bleeding under the skin while the animal is still alive (Fig. 2). Unless there are punctures, cuts or tears associated with the bruise, most bruising is sterile and would not contain pathogenic bacteria. The colour changes associated with bruises depend on the stage of the bruise. Fresh bruises are red from free blood under the skin and in the deeper tissues. Older bruises are black to blue, as the blood is reabsorbed and broken down. Older bruises change colours to green, then yellow, and then they fade. As blood breaks down, the pigments in it undergo the various colour changes. Blood pigments are not considered toxic and do not represent a food safety hazard.

Broilers are caught by the catch crew, loaded into crates and transported to the processing plant. During such processes, bruising and fractures may occur due to bad management or insufficient training (Fig. 3). Areas most frequently bruised are the breast, wings and legs (Fig. 4). The prevalence of red wing tips has been related to the severity and extent of wing flapping at hanging-on. Moreover, severe wing flapping before death will also lead to accelerated glycolysis of the breast muscle and thus decrease the meat quality.

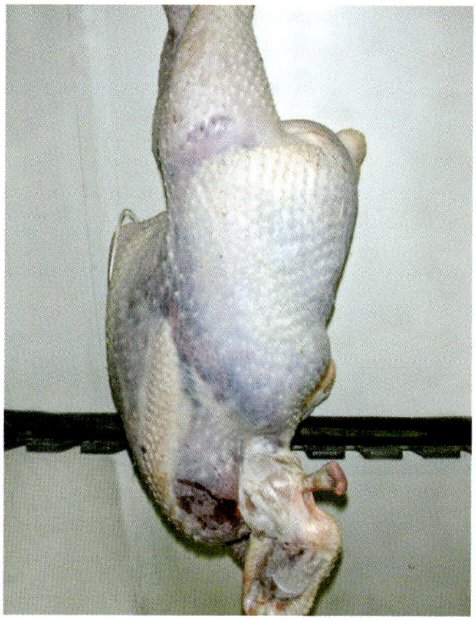

FIGURE 3. Extensive fresh bruising affecting most of the carcass. Broken vessels during catching or transport allowing a considerable amount of blood to spread under the skin. The plucking process might have exacerbated such spread of blood. Total rejection of the carcass is advised.

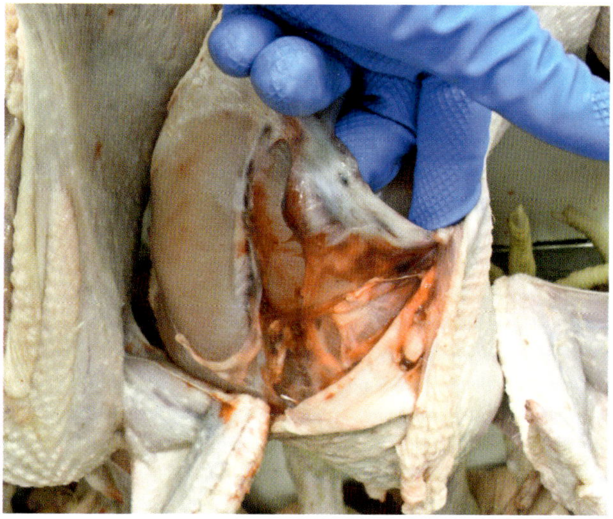

FIGURE 4. Proliferation of connective tissue affecting the breast area of a carcass. This condition is thought to be connected to a fast growth of the breast muscles and a permanent contact of the breast against the floor. When removed the underneath muscles appear clean and with no bruising. This condition should not be mistaken with bruising caused during catching or hanging and carcasses may be passed fit for human consumption once the relevant trimming has been carried out.

Responsibilities

Where bone fractures in poultry carcasses are detected at post-mortem inspection, disposition shall be in accordance with the following:

- Where the fracture is associated with a bruise, the fracture site and bruised tissue shall be trimmed off and condemned. With fractures that involve the bones of the wings and legs, the affected tissue shall be removed by incision through the first joint (or joints) outside the affected area (Fig. 5). In the case of a dislocated hip, without bruising, trimming is not required.
- Where the fracture is compound, i.e., the skin is penetrated, the fracture site and the surrounding tissue have to be trimmed off and condemned in a similar manner to that outlined above.
- Where the fracture is simple, without bruise or skin perforation, the affected portion may be approved for boning by either manual or mechanical means. In some cases, salvage may be possible by removing the affected area of fractured portions (Fig. 6), e.g., a simple fracture of the distal end of the tibia may be removed by cutting proximal to the fracture. In such a case, the affected part must be removed to the satisfaction of the inspector prior to approval of the remainder of the portion.

In those instances where trimming is impracticable, in other words where the carcass is extensively mutilated, then the carcass shall be condemned.

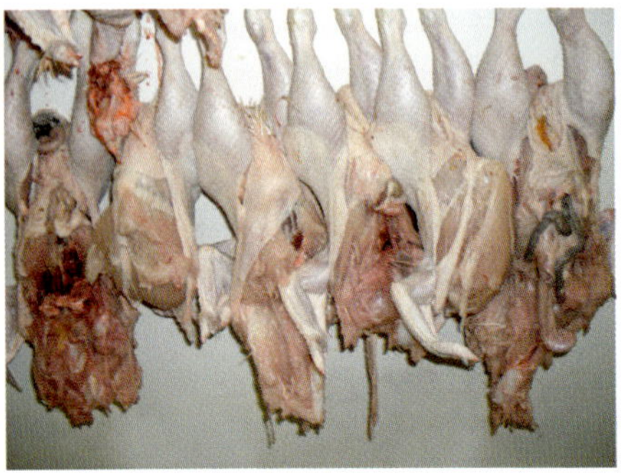

FIGURE 5. Extensive damage of the breast muscle and wings due to a malfunction of the plucking machine. Salvage of the legs possible.

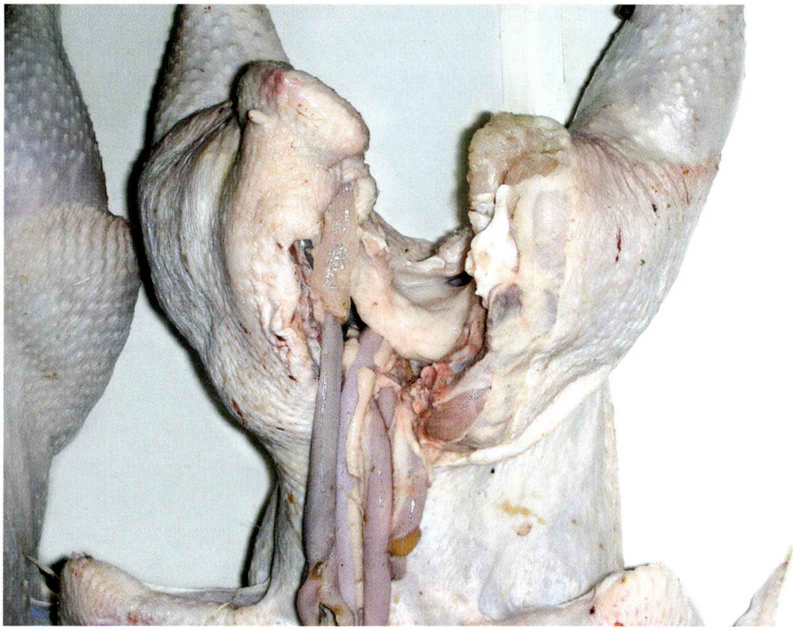

FIGURE 6. Damage to the pelvis. Salvage possible.

Bruising and fractures have serious animal welfare implications, carcass downgrading and yield loss.

There is no doubt that catching, loading, transportation, unloading and shackling may be painful, stressful and damaging processes. The rate and types of injury depend on many factors. Manual handling has been identified as the most potential source of injury and stress to the birds.

The inspector and veterinarian should always report any unnecessary suffering caused to the birds.

Meat fallen on the floor

The disposition of carcasses that fall on the floor from the automated lines must be left to the discretion of the veterinarian and the inspection team.

Hygienic handling of carcasses or portions, which have fallen on the floor, shall be conducted according to a procedure that has been validated as part of the operator's HACCP system. Such carcasses or portions shall be immediately removed from contact with the floor to avoid any risk of cross contamination. All visible contamination shall be removed by e.g. washing and/or trimming in an efficient yet sanitary fashion. After satisfactory removal of visible contamination, the carcass or portion shall be thoroughly rinsed with water. If salvage of the carcass or portion is not considered practicable, then condemnation needs to be considered. Salvage will depend mainly on the cleanliness of the place of the fall and the time spent in that location.

The place of the falls and their frequency should be recorded since this is valuable information to the inspection team and to the Food Business Operator. Corrective action to prevent recurrence may be required in those cases where contamination can compromise the wholesomeness of the final product.

References

Council Directive 2007/43 of 28 June 2007 laying down minimum rules for the protection of chickens kept for meat production. Official Journal L 182, 12/07/2007, p. 0019-0028. Available from http://eur-lex.europa.eu

Council Directive 93/119/EC of 22 December 1993 on the protection of animals at the time of slaughter or killing. Official Journal L 340, 31/12/1993, p. 0021-0034. Available from http://eur-lex.europa.eu

Council Regulation (EC) No 1099/2009 of 24 September 2009 on the protection of animals at the time of killing. Available from http://eur-lex.europa.eu

Council Regulation (EC) No 1/2005 of 22 December 2004 on the protection of animals during transport and related operations and amending Directives 64/432/EEC and 93/119/EC, and Regulation (EC) No 1255/97. Available from http://eur-lex.europa.eu

European Convention for the protection of animals for slaughter. Official Journal L 137, 02/06/1988, p. 0027-0038. Available from http://eur-lex.europa.eu

Manual for Official Controls of the Food Standards Agency. Aviation House, 125 Kingsway, London WC2B 6NH, United Kingdom. Available from http://www.food.gov.uk

Meat Industry Guide (MIG). Guide to Food Hygiene and other Regulations for the UK Meat Industry. Meat Hygiene and Veterinary Division, Food Standards Agency, 3rd floor, Aviation House, 125 Kingsway, London WC2B 6NH. Available from http://www.food.gov.uk

Meat chickens and breeding chickens. Code of recommendations for the welfare of livestock. DEFRA, Department for Environment, Food & Rural Affairs, United Kingdom. Available from http://www.food.gov.uk

Meat Hygiene Manual of Procedures. Canadian Food Inspection Agency. 1400 Merivale Road, Ottawa, Ontario, K1A 0Y9, Canada. Available from http://www.inspection.gc.ca

Regulation (EC) No 178/2002 of the European Parliament and of the Council of 28 January 2002 laying down the general principles and requirements of food law, establishing the European Food Safety Authority and laying down procedures in matters of food safety. Available from http://eur-lex.europa.eu

Regulation (EC) No 852/2004 of the European Parliament and of the Council of 29 April 2004 on the hygiene of foodstuffs. Available from http://eur-lex.europa.eu

Regulation (EC) No 853/2004 of the European Parliament and of the Council of 29 April 2004 laying down specific hygiene rules for food of animal origin. Available from http://eur-lex.europa.eu

Regulation (EC) No 854/2004 of the European Parliament and of the Council of 29 April 2004 laying down specific rules for the organisation of official controls on products of animal origin intended for human consumption. Available from http://eur-lex.europa.eu

The Welfare of Poultry at Slaughter or Killing Guidelines. Department for Environment, Food and Rural Affairs, Nobel House, 17 Smith Square, London SW1P 3JR. Available from http://www.food.gov.uk

Published by Servet editorial - Grupo Asís Biomedia S.L.